CHI GONG

Also by Paul Dong

Empty Force: The Power of Chi for Self-Defense and Energy Healing (with Thomas Raffill)

CHI GONG

The Ancient Chinese Way to Health

Paul Dong
and Aristide H. Esser, MD

BLUE SNAKE BOOKS

Published by Blue Snake Books

Blue Snake Books' publications are distributed by
North Atlantic Books   Cover photo by Paula Morrison
P.O. Box 12327   Cover design by Brad Greene
Berkeley, California 94712   Interior design by Eve Kirch

Printed in the United States of America

From the Marlowe & Company paperback edition, 1990

Chi Gong: The Ancient Chinese Way to Health is sponsored by the Society for the Study of Native Arts and Sciences, a nonprofit educational corporation whose goals are to develop an educational and cross-cultural perspective linking various scientific, social, and artistic fields; to nurture a holistic view of arts, sciences, humanities, and healing; and to publish and distribute literature on the relationship of mind, body, and nature.

North Atlantic Books' publications are available through most bookstores. For further information, call 800-733-3000 or visit our website at www.northatlanticbooks.com. or www.bluesnakebooks.com.

PLEASE NOTE: The creators and publishers of this book disclaim any liabilities for loss in connection with following any of the practices, exercises, and advice contained herein. To reduce the chance of injury or any other harm, the reader should consult a professional before undertaking this or any other martial arts, movement, meditative arts, health, or exercise program. The instructions and advice printed in this book are not in any way intended as a substitute for medical, mental, or emotional counseling with a licensed physician or healthcare provider.

Library of Congress Cataloging-in-Publication Data

Dong, Paul.
  Chi gong : the ancient Chinese way to health / by Paul Dong and Aristide H. Esser.
    p. cm.
  ISBN 978-1-58394-258-1
  1. Qi gong. I. Esser, Aristide H., 1930– II. Title.

RA781.8.D66 2008
613.7'1489—dc22
                                                          2008026131
                                                          CIP

1 2 3 4 5 6 7 8 9 UNITED 14 13 12 11 10 09 08

"Be imperturbable and the true chi will come to you;
concentrate the inner spirit and well-being will follow."

The Yellow Emperor's Classic of Internal Medicine

CONTENTS

ACKNOWLEDGMENTS

To many of our teachers and colleagues mentioned throughout this book, we owe a personal debt of gratitude. Our thanks go to Cyrus Lee, Robert Sampson, William Sacks, James Cappuccino, and Marcello Truzzi, who commented during the various stages of our manuscript. We are much obliged to Cynthia Lott Vogel for her drawing of figures 3-1, 3-2, 8-4, and 9-4. We also especially acknowledge our editorial adviser and literary agent John White, who originally suggested our collaboration. To Andy DeSalvo, our Paragon House editor, thank you for your patience and understanding.

For their early encouragement and unstinting attention to the work at hand, we must, too, thank Ada Reif Esser and Bruce Holbrook. Their contributions to the writing and editing of this text are invaluable.

FOREWORD

by Bruce Holbrook

Currently there is a potentially revolutionary transmission of Chinese medical ideas, practices, and materials to Europe and North America. This book focuses on what may be the most crucial concept to the success or failure of the West's attempt to adopt and make good use of these treasures. What I would like to say should prove useful to the reader who is not familiar with both the Chinese and American poles of this cultural transmission.

I began practicing chi gong—the cultivation and deliberate control of a higher form of vital energy—in 1969 in Taiwan, which was at that time the sector of China least transformed by Western civilization and hosting the greatest number per capita of traditional physicians and martial artists from all of the Chinese provinces. My teachers through 1974, Li Ts'an, Hsu Bei-Ying, and Chao Hsi-Ming (who is well-known among practitioners in America for his book of simple and potent chi gong longevity exercises), were all from Szechuan Province. The great Chinese civilization, colorful and exciting with its innumerable esoteric disciplines, was still to be felt as an integral whole into the 70s, although it was rapidly succumbing, via its own decay and Western political-economic pressures, to capitalist industrialization in Taiwan and Communist "up-rooting" on the

Mainland. Until the 70's, it was China experimenting with Western political and economic systems. Now, mainland and island are a cultural hybrid, no longer China.

Chinese medicine and martial arts, which include chi gong, no longer exist in their native context because that context is gone. Out of vital context, nothing survives *as it was*. Either it mutates to survive, or it is absorbed into something which is, as a whole, quite new. So far, the road has been one of mutation, and its positive or negative direction has yet to be determined. In the American desert the Chinese firecracker became the A-bomb, but in Turkish soil Virginia tobacco became more delicate and sweet.

As the authors here imply, and as I gathered from my limited success in communicating what I had learned in China, without intimate participatory experience in the native context, the true, or natively intended meanings of what one seeks to learn are difficult to apprehend fully or accurately. In addition, because of China's "hybrid" state, elements of what was once a balanced whole may be magnified or reduced in relative importance—as was acupuncture in the 1970s, in relation to (then virtually ignored) herbal medicine.

Chi gong in the genuine sense, then, along with the rest of Chinese medicine and martial arts, is a matter out of focus and in a state of mutation. Sensitive to this, the authors have taken great care to make explicit potentially misleading cross-cultural differences and to specify the concept of chi systematically. But this is not only a matter of translation, and here is where the reader comes in.

When we speak of something valuable, we speak, ultimately, of something beyond that metatool of humans, culture. We speak of something intrinsically valuable to human beings themselves, as distinguished, for example, from something valuable to a medical, political, or economic system. Humans everywhere become ill and seek health, and everywhere some humans seek to realize their potentials fully. Human beings from any culture ultimately judge their states of wellness or self-actualization with their senses, and, because the human senses and the human body are universal, the basic parameters of wellness, self-actualization, and judgement thereof are also universal. Chinese and American patients with the same diagnostics sense that they are better after taking the same herbal medicines, culturally conditioned interpretations notwithstanding. The "transporter-room" that beamed chi gong westward no longer exists, and chi gong is in an unfocused particle state; but the humans at the *receiving end* may, with care, bring the matter into focus, because the transmission has been from humans to humans.

Common to martial-arts varieties of chi gong is the set of exercises called Yi Jin, which means "using the tendons." It transforms shoulder and forearm tendons into whipcords, capable of great torque. After four years of practicing this discipline about forty-five minutes a day, I was able to visibly flood my arms and hands with blood (for heavier blows) simply by mentally preparing to strike. Then I could *immediately* deflate my arms by exhaling in a certain way. Only the coordination of breathing with conscious intention could produce these effects. Plainly, the chi can carry messages—instructions carried out metabolically. Sure enough, according to Chinese medical theory the chi moves the blood and yi (idea or ideational intent) can direct chi. But I did not know that when I began, and my chi gong teacher had not even specified the effects to be achieved. I intuitively realized those potentials, and the effects could be observed by anyone.

The preceding example illustrates the (typically Chinese) notion that, for everything invisible, or metaphysical, there is a visible, or otherwise sense-able correlate. As Dong and Esser remark, chi gong masters tend to be physically impressive. Where there is extraordinary presence of chi, there is also something extraordinary and observable in the gross physical sense, be it the delicacy of an accomplished acupuncturist's manipulations or the impact of a blow.

In the "Special Section on Chi" (chapter 1) I provide, on the basis of ordinary experiences and examples, logical demonstrations of the existence of chi and explanations of its different kinds. It will become apparent that what is most mystical about chi is Western science's systematic denial of sense evidence of its existence, and of logical implication of its vital primacy. Understanding this, and relying on their senses, American readers need only to remember that "only the balanced receiver can receive the balanced transmission." Esoteric Chinese concepts are all part of a spiritual and physical, or non-sensible and sensible, continuum that is in equilibrium. Americans tend either to be spiritually biased (and so to *believe*, despite sense data and logic to the contrary) or materially biased, practical, close-minded (and so to *disbelieve* despite sense data and logic to the contrary). Let us complete the continuum. Ideas can direct chi, but are ideas, then, the end of the continuum? Plainly, thought and imagination are tools, used by another part of ourselves, which has intention. This other part is spirit (*jing-shen*), that which freely chooses. Spirit produces ideational intent, which directs chi which in turn directs metabolism. Reciprocally, the gross physical body must become a vehicle conducive to any extraordinary chi activity. Through chi gong, "the copper coil becomes platinum," (i.e. conductivity increases), capillary capacity increases, and mass is added.

What is most important to remember about chi is that without recognition of its function and vital primacy there could be no true science of life, and so no genuine medicine. The concept of chi bridges the gap between what I have called "the two dead halves of Western medicine," psychotherapy and physical medicine. And the concept of chi is crucial to understanding any aspect of Chinese medicine. It is most opportune, therefore, that the authors have provided us with a book focusing on chi gong, that aspect of Chinese medical culture which most emphasizes chi.

As it's said, "The truth comes out in the end." The natural power of the concept of chi is healing the Western view of life and well-being not only on European and American soil, but also in mainland China, where the Marxist, antispiritual version of that view has been transplanted. Wishing to preserve China's medical treasures, yet to "destroy all the old superstitions," the postdynastic rulers of mainland China have been forced by vital reality to choose between the two by reclassifying chi as a "scientific" rather than "superstitious" concept. This book will present thorough documentation of this culturally and historically positive change. It is to be hoped that the next of a few more necessary steps, the recognition of the reality of spirit, and the freedom it requires, will also be taken. Toward that end, America, with its revolutionary culture of freedom, sets the best example for mainland China.

PREFACE

When we agreed to work together on this book, it was with the understanding that the experiences of Paul Dong during his intensive study and practice of chi gong throughout the past decade would be elaborated upon and, if necessary, clarified for the Western reader by Aristide H. Esser. We thought of it as a simple enough task, but soon realized that if we were to do justice to the ancient concept of chi, we would have to attempt a synthesis between traditional Chinese and modern Western thinking. Two problem areas became apparent: the nature of the subject per se and the political ramifications of chi gong's popular resurgence in the People's Republic of China.

First, one must realize that a full explanation of chi gong is impossible within modern Western thought. This does not mean that chi gong cannot be practiced in the West. It is possible to learn to improve and maintain one's health by following the rules for chi gong described in several chapters of this book and several other texts. However, to attain the full benefit of what Chinese savants call "mastering the chi," one would need to understand its ancient principles and discipline oneself to follow *its* logic. And in these areas some of the most basic assumptions of the modern Western worldview have to be set aside. Many of the concepts we discuss in this book help to explain the apparently incredible claims of chi gong experts (for example, that the practice of chi gong can cure cancer or enable the chi gong master to influence someone's biological functions by simply pointing a finger), but these concepts originated in an ancient Eastern worldview.

Second, the modern Chinese history of chi gong reflects its role in the internal politics of mainland China, as this country tries to regain a major role in world affairs. Chi gong and its major related practices, such as acupuncture and the martial arts, do not fit well into the plans of a nation trying to modernize, especially when that nation espouses the Western materialistic philosophy of Marxism. After the establishment of the People's Republic of China in 1949, only the demonstration of the efficacy of traditional Chinese medicine during the fighting years of the Red Revolutionary Army, combined with China's dire need for medical care, forced Mao to exhort both Chinese practitioners of Western medicine (roughly 12,000 at that time) and doctors of traditional Chinese medicine (numbering 370,000 and thus the great majority[1]) to work together.[2] Also, both old and new medicine were given equal status in education, practice, and research. However, leading Chinese government health advisers, including the American doctor George Hatem,[3] favored Western medicine, as shown by the present two-to-one ratio between Chinese Western trained doctors and practitioners of traditional medicine.

Ironically, while acupuncture gained recognition early in the seventies, chi gong, the cornerstone of ancient Chinese healing practices, including acupuncture, gained prominence only recently after a national uproar over what China calls *exceptional human functions,* or what in Western terms would be called psychic phenomena. We review the recent history of chi gong in chapter 10, and point to this heated public debate as indicative of the problems encountered when writing about what were, until recently, considered esoteric practices.

Within, China the deep-seated philosophical clash between Chinese traditional science and Western thought, and the lingering political ambivalence about the value of chi gong, have affected the credibility of modern scientific research into the effects of chi. Any proposed joint Sino-U.S. medical research effort seems to flounder once conditions for the experiments are spelled out, much as happens with parapsychological research in the West. The authors have no doubt that failures in arriving at empirical research agreements will continue as long as the underlying differences in the Chinese and Western worldviews are not taken into account and, at the very least, articulated. We will try to contribute to a mutually acceptable framework for chi gong research by exploring basic concepts throughout this book and by providing a brief review of possible Western approaches to chi research in the final chapter.

We ask that you approach the subject of chi gong with an open mind, with the attitude of a cautious yet curious explorer. We hope that you will read this book literally as you would watch a film or a play, to look at the whole story and not relate only to those parts with which you can agree. It is not necessary for you to be convinced by everything we have to say in order for this book to broaden your horizons. For we believe it is important not only to search for the tangible benefits of age-old non-Western traditions dealing with health, but also to explore the consequences of traditional Chinese knowledge for modern thought in this age of global interdependence.

The concept of chi conveys a message which lies in the relationships between the effects of chi presented and their therapeutic usage. The message deals with health.

Today, whether one is a layperson or a health professional, one cannot help but notice that, because of the myriad medical technologies in ever increasing areas of specialization driving the modern Western health delivery system, there is a growing dissatisfaction with our health care. Modern medicine appears to depend more on the knowledge of detailed mechanisms than of the whole person.

This spurs our search for a focus in becoming whole and healthy. According to ancient Chinese wisdom, the unifying principle of health as symbolized by chi gong is the way to well-being and longevity.

Paul Dong and Aristide H. Esser

Notes

1. According to Edgar Snow in *Red China Today* (New York: Random House, 1970), 300.

2. This forced collaboration has brought about at least one major breakthrough: the use of acupuncture anaesthesia. In several types of major operations this form of anaesthesia has been proven to be safer and have fewer side effects than conventional (chemical) anaesthesia.

3. How Dr. Hatem gained the confidence of Mao in 1936 is recounted in Edgar Snow's authoritative book *Red Star over China* (New York: Random House, 1938; rev. ed., New York: Grove Press, 1968). Dr. Ma Hai-de (Hatem's Chinese name) for fifty years, until his death in 1988, helped guide the health policies of Communist China. Among his prodigious accomplishments, he is credited with eradicating many infectious diseases, for which he received the prestigious Albert Lasker Public Service Award in 1986 in the U.S. Because of Dr. Ma Hai-de's immense experience in Chinese health practices, Aristide Esser was surprised to learn of his reservations regarding the theory of traditional Chinese medicine during a 1984 dinner meeting.

Introduction

One sunrise in 1984, in October when the early mornings of South China are still hot, a group of twenty Americans, between the ages of fifty and sixty, set out to travel by bike from Guangzhou to Conghua. Twenty kilometers later, six were too exhausted to go on, so they laid their bikes at the roadside and took a rest. After about fifteen minutes, their guide and interpreter Luo Yao-ming came over to urge them not to spend too much time resting, but the six people remained immobile even after half an hour. The driver of their support bus became impatient and proposed to transport them and their bikes to Conghua. "Wait a minute," said Luo, "perhaps I could get them to take to the road again." He then took them into the bus, one by one, and gave each one a chi[1] gong treatment for about twenty seconds. Miraculously, all six regained their strength, mounted their bicycles and proceeded to their destination. Later they told a reporter, from whom Paul Dong heard this story, that it was only when Luo applied what they now understood to be chi to their Yong Quan point (an acupuncture point in the foot) that they felt invigorated. Luo is a young chi gong master who from the age of five received his training from his grandmother.

Chi gong is an approach to mind/body exercises, following ancient

Chinese tradition, which has become immensely popular in the People's Republic of China since 1982. Chi gong was long neglected except by an elite, comprised primarily of Confucian scholars, Taoists, Buddhist priests, and students of ancient medicine and martial arts, who carried on the practice. Few of the generation growing up during the Communist period knew anything about it and it was not until 1979 that chi gong was brought to the attention of the general public (as we will discuss in chapter 10). This ancient practice has been rediscovered, and as a result there is at present a veritable chi gong craze throughout China. In Beijing alone there are over three hundred thousand practitioners, including the one hundred chi gong team members of the *People's Daily*, China's leading newspaper with a circulation of eleven million.

As Dong learned during his many visits to mainland China, and as Esser was told in August 1984 when visiting the Beijing Institute of Traditional Chinese Medicine, there are myriad chi phenomena, divided broadly into two categories: hard and soft.

Instances of *hard chi gong* include breaking steel rods with one's foot, splitting bricks by hand or breaking a piece of marble by running into it headfirst, resisting a knife or sword thrust to the body, surviving without harm a car being driven over one's body, and injuring someone with merely a finger. The photographs below demonstrate the hard chi gong practitioners' ability to prevent their skin from being perforated by sharp objects. Such performances of hard chi gong are common in China; in fact, they constitute a means of earning a livelihood for itinerant entertainers.

Soft chi gong serves different purposes. Mastering it would enable one not only to prevent or overcome illness but also to cure certain ailments in others. The latter type of therapy rests on the principle of shifting energy from oneself to the patient and thereby enhancing his/her energetic condition. Naturally, the chi energy from the donor is not inexhaustible and must be acquired by the daily practice of chi gong, as described in chapters 8 and 9.

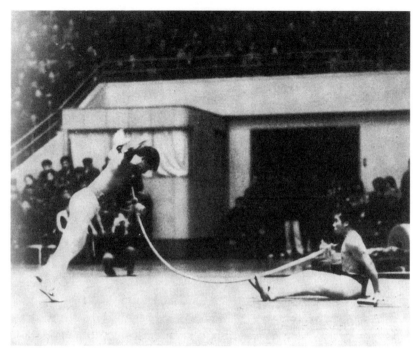

Hard chi gong: "The throat drilling silver spear." Each performer sticks one of the sharp ends of a double-pointed spear at his throat and bends it by pushing while remaining unharmed.

The purported nature and source of chi energy are ignored by Western science and medicine. At this time there appears to be no way in which the Chinese concept of chi can be expressed adequately in Western medical terms. But as we will show, chi gong, as an ancient Chinese way to health, is quite accessible to Westerners in some forms. The current, very popular techniques are not difficult to learn and lead to results that not only have been observed for thousands of years but also seem to withstand the scrutiny of modern testing methods. Above all, they fulfill the medical dictum of *primum non nocere,* that is, "first, do no harm."

Chi is a universal force which is part of any life-form. It can be strengthened in humans by certain practices under the general name

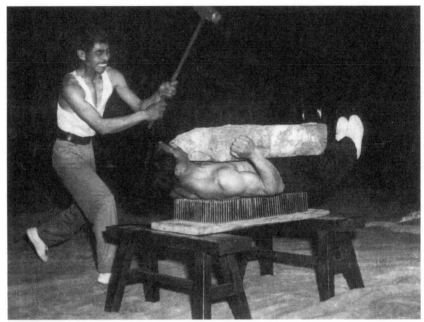

Hard chi gong: "Being hammered in a bed of nails." The performer remains unscathed notwithstanding the severe insults to the body. (Photo courtesy of Wang Jia Lin.)

of chi gong. The Chinese believe that we need chi as we need blood. Codified more than two thousand years ago in *The Yellow Emperor's Classic of Internal Medicine*,[2] the equivalent of the medical writing of Hippocrates, the ancient Chinese determined that there were two separate circulations in the body. They discovered the first, the circulation of blood, thousands of years before William Harvey did in England. The second, and the one of importance to us, was described as the circulation of chi, an energy pumped by the lungs to circulate in invisible body tracts. Their "entire view of the body and its functioning was that of a dual circulation theory of blood (which was yin) and chi (which was yang). The two were interrelated," as Robert Temple reports in *The Genius of China*.[3] Just as we may experience dysfunction when our blood stagnates or does not circulate properly throughout the body, so our functions may fail when the circulation of chi is faulty.

Luo determined that the circulation of chi in the tired bicyclists needed activation and did so by influencing an acupuncture point in the foot. We will discuss the importance of the age-old Chinese wisdom pertaining to the flow of energy through the body and why the Chinese call chi the universal life energy. We will teach you how the flow of chi can be regulated by simple exercises, and how certain chi gong practitioners become capable of transferring its benefits to other people. Above all, we will show how chi gong can complement and strengthen the results of Western health care.

Notes

1. Long spelled *ch'i* or *chi* (Wade-Giles romanization system), but in the modern pinyin romanization system rendered *qi*. For reasons of its familiar usage, we retain *chi* and *chi gong*, making an exception to our use of the modern pinyin spellings in this book.

2. I. Veith, trans., *The Yellow Emperor's Classic of Internal Medicine*, 2d ed. (Berkeley: Univ. of California Press, 1972). In this book, referred to as *The Emperor's Classic*.

3. Robert Temple, *The Genius of China: 3,000 Years of Science, Discovery, and Invention* (New York: Simon and Schuster, 1986).

1

What Is Chi Gong?

The function of the tract-channel system of the human body is to promote a normal passage (circulation) of the blood and the ch'i.

—*The Yellow Emperor's Classic of Internal Medicine*

Chi gong (also spelled *chi kung* and *qi gong*) is an ancient Chinese system of "breathing" or "vital energy" mind control exercises. It has a remarkably positive effect on health. It can help prevent and cure diseases, increase strength, resist premature senility, and ensure long life. In ancient China it was called a method for "warding off diseases and prolonging life."

Traditional Chinese medicine (TCM) holds that the person is a unity in which illness is caused by an imbalance of the vital force and the body fluids (blood). The inclusive concept of balancing, complementing, and contradictory actions of life forces derives from the predominant Chinese philosophy of the opposites of *yin* (negative) and *yang* (positive) that are ultimately integrated in the universal force, symbolized in the *tai-ji* diagram (see fig. 1-1).

The *tai-ji* symbolizes the Chinese belief in the absence of absolutes, which can be verbalized as "what is, is also what is not," a statement that would make little sense to the Westerner. Be that as it may, from this fundamental Chinese understanding of the polarity and complimentary of the universe comes the belief that in white there must always be black, and vice versa. The acceptance of a basic

1

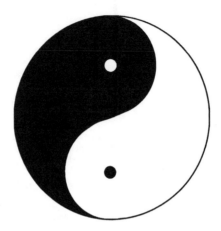

The *tai ji* diagram with intertwined *yang* and *yin*.

completeness automatically brings with it the possibility of restoration of balance and harmony in anything, including human life. This can be achieved by reconciling or relaxing the "antagonisms" between polar axes of tension. For the maintenance of health, among the most important polarities to be balanced are: *yin-yang* (female-male, dark-light, etc.), *piao-li* (outer-inner), *leng-je* (hot-cold), and *hsü-shih* (empty-solid).

The literal translation of the Chinese character for chi is *air* or *breath*. One might immediately think of the air we breathe, and while this is correct to some extent, the Chinese consider air to be a mixture of chi and gases. According to ancient Chinese metaphysics, the first meaning of chi is "configurational energy,"[1] which underlies all of the organization in the universe. Further, chi is the primal matrix of creation from which spring the *yin* and *yang* forces that give rise to substance and material forms. What concerns us here is the part of chi that is life energy, or the universal force that animates all living things providing vitality to matter.

Chi gong is the collective name for many ancient Chinese exercises that allow us to gain control over chi, the life energy distributed through invisible channels in our body. It is the maintenance of the balanced distribution of chi that guarantees health and well-being. One of the ways to understand this is to familiarize oneself with the representation of chi's invisible channels, or tracts, by the "meridians" used in acupuncture. To be able to treat an illness, the acupuncturist must (according to custom) be oriented by twelve to fourteen lines (meridians) visualized on the body surface. This is an easy way to memorize which acupuncture points are related to specific organ functions. The meridians are not themselves conduits for the chi energy, because the channels are within the body, not superficially on the skin. But insertion of acupuncture needles to certain depths at the acupoints will assist in balancing the circulation of chi (discussed in chapter 3).

Even if we are not willing to subscribe to the philosophy of the *tai-ji* or the Chinese belief that chi gong exercises are related to an awareness of the needs and wishes of our body, we may want to practice them. In the West, we acknowledge many self-regulating balancing mechanisms which are conveyed through our autonomous nervous system and of which we are rarely conscious. For instance, a pregnant woman may crave certain foods that will provide her with needed nutrients and minerals; when our blood-sugar level is low we may feel faint or irritable, and try to help ourselves by eating or drinking. But, according to traditional Chinese understanding, chi gong exercises *deliberately* call upon the *yin* and *yang* forces to bring self-regulating balance to the body. To accept the possibility of this type of control over our (unconscious) physiological mechanisms, we must begin with an understanding of the basic concepts of "chi" and "gong." In doing so, we will use the concepts of Chinese scientific thinking, with the realization that these may be unacceptable or even incomprehensible to Western thinking. Wherever possible, we will insert Western concepts that may convey similar meaning.[2]

However, let's keep in mind that a direct translation from ancient Eastern to modern Western thinking is impossible at this time, and that our attempts at mutual understanding are only tentative (as summarized in chapter 13).

The recognition of a general life energy is universal. In Western thought there has been the ancient concept of the soul, the vital principle of the body. Among the better known contemporary examples of life energy are the Polynesian mana, the Indian prana or kundalini, and, in the eighteenth century, Mesmer's "animal magnetism." In this century Henri Bergson, the French Nobel laureate philosopher, conceived of the "vital impulse" (*elan vital*), as part of the doctrine of "vitalism," which holds that a force peculiar to living organisms controls their form and development.

Perhaps we might call chi the "breath of life." As Bruce Holbrook's *shih-fu* (teaching father)[3] put it, "Ch'i without body has no place to be-at, body without ch'i does not live."[4] It is the latter chi that is mastered in such familiar practices as *tai ji quan* and the Japanese *aikido*.

According to Dr. Cyrus Lee, who teaches "psychology of consciousness" at Edinboro State College in Pennsylvania, "Qi and Qigong must be rather experienced than defined." He quotes Master Guo Lin (whose cancer therapy will be described in chapter 5) as follows: "Qi cannot be seen by your eyes and cannot be grasped by your hands. But a Qigong master is different from ordinary people, because he can apparently realize something moving and promulgating in his body, something like the electric current circulating within you and making some tingling feelings."[5]

According to research by Chinese scientists, chi gong masters may be able to transfer different kinds of chi. When measured by sophisticated apparatus such transfers have been shown to contain infrared radiation, static electricity, and particle currents from magnetic fields—neutrons, beta rays, and infrasonics. And from studying the effects of chi on the human body, these scientists have concluded that it is comprised of both a kind of informational message and its carrier, with the carrier definitely acknowledged to be a material substance. As Xu Hong-zhang and Zhao Yong-jie from the Institute of High Energy Physics in Beijing put it:

> The Chi is considered today somewhat like radiation in modern physics, but there is a difference in that the Chi concept emphasizes not only an energy aspect, but also an information aspect. Thus it is emphasized that Chi makes it possible for separated bodies to transmit information as well as energy to one another.[6]

Thus the *chi* in *chi gong* is not simply the oxygen inhaled or the carbon dioxide exhaled; it is a complex energy substance, fundamental to life itself. It is understandable that, given the importance of chi for the myriad functions of the living organism, there exist many forms of chi. It may appear quite confusing to try to follow the Chinese distinctions between many different types and states of chi energy, and many might deem it unnecessary as well. However, the proliferation of meanings for what we might be inclined to call simply "the life force" may be understood if we think of the need for special knowledge in different cultures. For instance, the Eskimo have many different terms for snow and ice. To the Eskimo, precise differentiation between wet driven snow and light dry snow, or between solid ice with or without cracks and ice floes, may prove a matter of life and death. Since ancient times, the Chinese distinguish many types of chi as they pertain to health and well-being under different circumstances. As we could not do justice to a description of all those forms and aspects of chi energy which are important for this book, we are grateful to Professor Holbrook for writing about the implications of the concept of chi in the "Special Section on Chi" provided at the end of this chapter. What follows here is a discussion of the observed effects of chi gong, including several brief descriptions of chi which are necessary to understand this discussion.

Chi gong practitioners generally call the chi they summon up in training "true chi" or "inner chi," to distinguish it, for instance, from the chi they inhale and exhale in normal breathing and the "external chi" they may be able to emit. Chinese medicine considers the "true chi" required by human bodies as the primary activating force of human life; therefore the quickening of chi in chi gong is training of the "true chi."

The goal of chi gong is to make the true chi circulate regularly and strongly in the human body. This achievement is a basic form of *gong fu* (or *kung fu*). The Chinese character *gong*, which basically means *work* or *self-discipline*, symbolizes physical prowess and its manifestation in the natural movements of the body. It also means merit, achievement, efficacy, or simply "good result," which leads to "the art of mastering." Although chiefly associated with the martial arts, *gong fu* may take the form of many results other than fighting skills and self-defense.

The time taken for training reflects the will and determination of the student. To "go fishing for three days and dry the nets for two"— in other words, to be unable to persevere in training—is not the way to obtain desired results. Persistence is absolutely necessary in chi gong training. The quality of training relates directly to the result and skill obtained. *Gong* is also called "the cultivation of the true chi." When true chi is developed the body becomes strong. Training for true chi should be carried out in three respects: "to direct jing chi[7] by breathing, to safeguard the spirit independently, and to unify the muscles and the flesh" (*The Emperor's Classic*).[8] These are the same as the training of "breath," "thought" and "body parts."

Chi gong practiced to master the manipulation of vital energy is crucial to Chinese traditional medicine. Masters[9] of this practice (originally Taoist or Buddhist monks) control their chi and are able to direct it through any part of their body (*nei chi*) as well as external to their body (*wei chi*) and thereby perform exceptional human functions (EHF), as recounted in chapters 7 and 10.

Methods of chi gong training differ from school to school. There are five major traditions of Chinese training in chi gong: Taoist, Buddhist, Confucian, medical, and martial arts. In actual practice, many of these schools overlap. The Taoist school lays emphasis on training both the body and the mind. It is called the "dual cultivation of nature and life" because it stresses the relation between the individual and the (ultimately cosmic) environment. The Buddhist school gives precedence to the cultivation of the mind and the moral will. The Confucian school emphasizes setting the conceptual mind right, honesty of higher thought, and altruism. The object is to obtain rest, steadiness, and tranquility. The medical school of chi gong training aims chiefly at curing illness; at the same time it considers hygiene and the prolongation of life. The martial arts school fosters strengthening of the body to resist attack and teaches striking at the enemy in self- or other-protection. Some of the chi gong methods are extremely rigorous and even dangerous. For instance, martial chi gong training may entail risking one's own life for the sake of health (safety) and the longevity of others.

Some Western-trained Chinese scientists claim proof of the existence of some chi manifestations, and its physical forms are being examined by scientific means. For instance, it is said that a stream of energy has been observed shooting from the fingertips of a chi gong master when projecting chi. Chinese scientists have concluded that this stream of energy is electromagnetic. This energy can cause physiological changes in others. For instance, Que Ash-ui, a Shanghai chi gong master, can make someone feel heavy, swollen, numb, and hot by projecting his chi. Master Lin Hou-sheng can produce surgically useful anaesthesia, under which a patient can undergo an operation lasting up to four hours. Master Zhao Wei can move something as far as three feet away when he projects his chi.

According to Professor Xie Huan-zhang of Beijing Industrial

College, chi effects have been successfully detected with instruments. Among chi's reported manifestations are low-frequency amplitude-modulated infrared radiation (the most common effect), low-frequency magnetic fields, particle-flow signals, infrasound,[10] and ion streams, including visible light and superfaint luminescence. These physical manifestations are capable of producing both physiological and healing effects on the diseased body. Is this due to energy or something else? Some Chinese scientists believe that healing with a chi gong master's external chi is nothing more than the effect of infrared heat waves, similar to physiotherapy's "diathermy." True, a chi gong master's external chi in most cases does contain infrared radiation, but according to repeated measurements, the power is only several tenths of a microwatt, while the power of the radiation energy used in physiotherapy is from tens to hundreds of watts, that is to say several tenths of a kilowatt. The microwatt (10^{-6} watt) and the kilowatt (10^3 watt) differ by many orders of magnitude. Thus, in comparison, the amount of heat-energy released by a chi gong master is extremely slight as compared to an infrared light. And yet, the healing power of the chi gong master appears much greater than the energy from the infrared radiation given in physiotherapy.

As the above shows, known and measurable physical energy cannot be the main factor in the ability of the chi gong master to produce physiological and therapeutic effects. Then what does enable chi to have the striking effects recognized for thousands of years in traditional Chinese medicine? In order to answer this question, its mechanism would have to be studied in depth. The results of measurements are controversial but abound in intriguing facts. For instance, infrasound with very low energy can damage the body's internal organs, even inducing fatal injuries. There is research being conducted into building infrasonic weapons. It is possible that a slight amount of energy can produce damage by evoking resonance in living tissue. In that case, the effects of infrasound would come mainly from its wave properties and its fluctuation, not from its energy level. This is similar to the capability of infrared chi radiation to produce physiological and healing effects because of its wave properties and fluctuation, not because of its intensity.

The infrared radiation released, for instance, from the palm of most people does not produce healing effects. But in the case of a chi gong master there appears to be an information content added to the release of chi, which is responsible for the effects on the recipient's body. Professor Xie Huan-zhang of the Beijing Industrial College (from whose book *The Scientific Basis of Chi Gong*[11] the above material was derived) reasons that the external chi of a master produces some response or resonance in the body of the receiver, which in turn produces the physiological or healing effect. Figures 1-2 and 1-3 illustrate the difference between the unmodulated infrared radiation of a person who has never practiced chi gong and the strongly differentiated infrared radiation from Master Zhao Guang

Research has shown that the properties of external chi produced by various chi gong masters differ according to their methods of chi gong training. Through this research, the presence of electrical energies in biological organisms has been generally accepted in science.[12] The human body can be considered a large bioelectrical field, which radiates low energy, the total strength perhaps adding up to an electric current required to power a color television set. Electrocardiograms (ECG, EKG—measurement of heart waves), electro- and magneto-encephalograms (composites of brain waves by EEG—electroencephalography—machines and by the SQUID—superconducting quantum interference device), electromagnetic scanners (whose images are made possible by computer-powered signal detection) are all witness to the fact that the activities of our organs, including the thinking activity of the brain, have bioelectrical consequences.

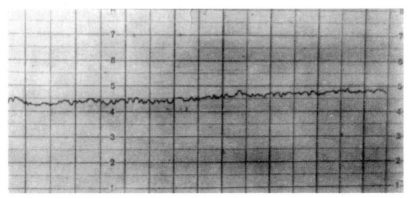

Signal obtained from an ordinary person tested for infrared emission. (*Photo courtesy of Zhou Wen Bin.*)

Master Zhao Guang holds his palm one meter in front of an infrared-ray detection device. Note the marked increase in the signal as compared to that of the ordinary person in Figure 1–2. (*Photo courtesy of Zhou Wen Bin.*)

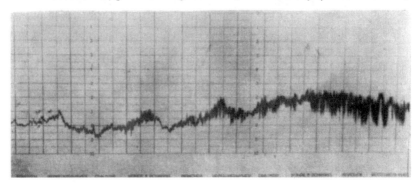

Scientists at the Space-Medico-Engineering Research Institute in Beijing, under the direction of Chung Jiang-xiang, have tested the human body's electromagnetic (EM) field. They suggest:

> The human body's potential can be divided into two parts: one part is hidden inside the body and is a dynamic interrelated network, such as the network of the meridians in traditional Chinese medicine. The other part of the potentials expresses itself in radiating forms, becoming energy fields, in all the different kinds of information sent out by chi gong masters. The potentials of the human body fall under the influence of the surrounding environment, and also under the influence of the condition of the body itself. When the body is sick, energy fields in particular areas go through changes. A person's spiritual condition and mental state both influence the energy field. Every person has the power to transmit as well as to receive energy field information signals. However, this power differs between people. Certain people, such as chi gong masters, children with inborn psychic abilities, and so on, possess extremely strong powers (levels of sensitivity) for transmitting and receiving energy field information signals. Others can greatly strengthen their levels of sensitivity through training, such as those who develop psychic powers by practicing chi gong. [13]

Furthermore, these scientists stated:

> The majority of human body potentials express themselves by means of electromagnetic energy fields. Every activity of the life system is accompanied by electric phenomena. Such physiological processes as nerve conduction, the beating of the heart, the activity of the brain, tensing of the muscles, and secretion from the glands will all give rise to corresponding electrical change. [14]

Indeed, the electrocardiograms, electroencephalograms, electroretinograms, and electrographs of many different organs record the electrical signal changes.

The role of magnetic fields in nature has increasingly drawn scientific attention. It is now an accepted fact that many animals have the ability to sense magnetic fields. For instance, in their long-distance migration, birds apparently use the earth's magnetic field for navigation. That humans may have retained this sensitivity to the earth's magnetic field has been shown in controlled experiments by Robin Baker in England. He reported on blindfolded volunteers transported to randomly chosen locations where they were able to indicate the direction of their point of origin and the directions of the compass. [15]

Beyond the earth's magnetic field, more and more physicists and medical specialists have taken an interest in the magnetic field of the human body. Some people are able to see auras surrounding the human figure and around magnets. Gu Han-seng of China's Institute of Nuclear Energy Research in Shanghai has measured the magnetic information produced by chi gong masters. In that city, Dong personally witnessed two chi gong masters, Chong Wan-yi and Bei Ji-jing, control the motions of a compass needle with their palms. Dong believes that the magnetic energy is strongest in the center of the hands of chi gong practitioners. He states:

> The final point I wish to raise here is that when I use chi to push people backwards without touching them, what is felt by the "target" person is a force-field effect. This field is clearly produced by the body electromagnetic energy field. When others use chi to push me without touching me, I will also feel the force field. Moreover, a person trained to produce external chi will feel an attraction between the palms after having these face each other for a while. [16]

Purportedly, chi gong training can activate and generate all the bodily energies, of which bioelectrical energy is most readily measured. However, traditional Chinese science, as we have shown before, considers chi an organized fundamental energy substance with many presently unmeasurable aspects. For instance, a superior chi gong master, by directing chi to the head, can break a block of marble by running into it headfirst; by directing chi to the body, the master can resist the penetration of iron spikes under pressure.[17] And it is claimed that the willfully manipulated movement of chi within the body of a chi gong master massages the internal organs, breaking down the congestions, clearing the blood vessels, and adjusting physiological functions so as to provide resistance to illness and ensure health. Unfortunately, none of these results of mastery of internal chi can be measured.

When chi gong training reaches a higher level, some special and peculiar functions of the human body are brought into play (supersensitive persons with specially sensitive meridians or energy passageways may reach this stage more quickly). In this case the trainee will not only be able to issue external chi, but will be able to see auras around people and practice telepathy or other exceptional human functions, as the Chinese call psychic powers.

It can be seen that chi gong has many implications for medicine and for the maintenance of good health. What about its application in martial arts, or *wu shu?* Here chi gong can have serious consequences. In *wu shu, dim mak* (Cantonese), or *dim yue,* a kind of rapidly applied hard chi gong, can be fatal. This "touch of death" involves using a fingertip to apply chi at another person's acupuncture points, and this may cause instant numbness or loss of consciousness. Depending on the force and place of application, injuries or death may result. If the master merely wants to teach someone a lesson and applies it lightly, the victim will recover within fifteen minutes. If the master applies it heavily, the victim may be seriously maimed or even killed. Such action combines chi gong with *wu shu* and the force of application is controlled by the power of the will. Of course, when shooting at the acupoint, timing and split-second action are required. Such manipulative skills are not easy to master and are said to require more than ten years of practice. *Dim mak* is impressively powerful, but it requires physical contact. Another type of chi gong, called *fa sheh gong* (projecting art), can cause death without body contact, even from a distance of ten feet. It resembles the effect of photon guns in science fiction or lasers in modern physics.

As we will discuss in chapter 9, the chi gong master may simply direct chi energy to the finger or project it from the center of the palm (the thunder, or magic, palm). This level of skill requires more than twenty years of training without skipping a day's practice—at least an hour daily and best done between three and five in the morning. In China, a country with a billion people, only a few chi gong masters have attained this high level.

Special Section on Chi, By Bruce Holbrook

The concept of chi is confusing to Western readers, not because it is a difficult one, but because our own culture stands in the way.

Occidental civilization is based on certain religious and philosophical premises which invite false translation of chi and related concepts. For example, our philosophy forces a choice between two fundamental levels of reality, which in the Chinese worldview are but a single one. That historically recent epistemological expression of our civilization, science, forcefully fights against comprehension of a single reality. Throughout this section, therefore, "science" and related terms such as "physical," are used within quotation marks when they refer to Western concepts. This may promote correction of the false, but very widespread, ethnocentric assumption that Western science is the only form of science.

Our "science" is firmly based on inanimate models and data-recording devices, whereas chi (in the central sense of this book) is intimately related to *distinctively* animate phenomena and cultivated human sensing. An additional problem is that Western science—especially "medical science"—has become dogmatic, so that it rejects any logical conclusion which lies outside its paradigm. The prevailing attitude is: If we can't deal with it in our terms, it does not exist, because only our terms are valid. Cultural anthropologists call such systematic ignorance "ethnocentrism"—being confined, unaware of the confinement, by one's own culture.

Given such widespread ethnocentrism, it is only natural therefore that Western thinking beyond the scope of "science" has surrounded chi with a mystical aura, while "scientific thinking" has reduced and deformed the concept into something manageable in its own terms. Such terms are untrue to the original concept and reality of chi. Beyond that there is a natural difficulty with distinctions among different kinds of chi. This can give rise to the impression that Chinese thinkers indulged in unnecessary conceptual multiplication to compensate for their own weaknesses in natural-scientific understanding. Nothing could be further from the truth.

Because Western thinkers do think in "scientific terms," much of the following clarification and simplification of the chi concept uses them. But the reader should understand that this is to approach chi from the odd angle obliged by our conceptual repertoire, and that this is not by any means an attempt to "scientifically" prove or explain the existence of chi. The scope of "science" is too narrow to provide adequately for such an attempt.

I think the best way to begin is with a distinction between two basic kinds of chi in living organisms, *original* and *formative*, as variables which 'fill holes' left by Western science. In this way cultural-conceptual confusion is precluded. It is primarily a matter of common sense.

I begin with a personal experience of a kind the reader may find easy to replicate or remember. As an adolescent frequently in front of a mirror, I noticed that when I was in a good mood my hair would stay combed, but when I was depressed it would fall out of place. (As I learned years later, *li*, in the medical expression *li chi*—to organize the chi—is the same as *li* in *li tou-fa*—to comb the hair.) Plainly, this phenomenon involved an electromagnetic (EM) field, but, I reasoned, there must be some mood-related phenomenon, other than or more than mood, which was responsible for the EM energy and fluctuations in the energy level of the field. I could envision my body as an EM coil, my hair as iron filings forming a pattern partly determined by the EM field around the coil—but what was the battery or generator of electricity? The answer to that lies in a recognition of Western science's illogical treatment of the matter of life and death.

Western science recognizes, via its metering devices, that the living organism possesses an EM field. And both meters and Kirlian photography show that the field extends beyond the "physical" (visible, palpable) boundary of the body. But "science" proposes that this field is biologically secondary, an effect produced by the biochemical substance of the body. This seems logical enough until we ask: What is the difference between a living human (or animal or plant) and a corpse, and why? What causes fetuses to be formed? What causes living tissue to regenerate? To these questions science has no answers that are not circular or evasive in logic.

The differences between a living human being and a corpse are that the former has an EM field and movement (together called "bioenergy") and neutral chemical acidity, whereas the latter lacks an EM field, does not move, and is highly acidic. Three possible implied explanations for the changes between the living and dead can be stated in the form of propositions: (1) absence of bioenergy is an effect of altered biochemistry (the Western scientific proposition); (2) altered biochemistry and exhaustion of bioenergy are effects of a third factor; (3) altered biochemistry is an effect of exhaustion of bioenergy (the Chinese scientific proposition).

(1) The Western Scientific Proposition This first explanation is the one used by modern science, and as we'll see it is an illogical and a let's-pull-ourselves-up-by-the-bootstraps type of thinking. Altered biochemistry requires an alterer. Chemical substances cannot in themselves account for the alteration. That is, given the formulas for these substances and the fact of their replenishment from blood, no change is predictable. As far as *biochemical* description can go—the biochemical composition of cells and fluids—the structure of the body of a healthy young person is the same as that of one who is about to die of old age.[18]

Let's further examine the western scientific proposition in order to approach the reality and nature of chi. From the perspective of a biochemist, it might be proposed that the independent variable is simply entropy—the "negative force" which diffuses concentrations of energy. The body is like a battery: its biochemicals are like the chemicals in a battery, its energetic conduit corresponds to the copper coil connecting the battery's poles, and its totality of energy represents the electromagnetism of the coil. The battery has a lifetime, even if it is recharged, at the end of which its chemical structures alter and render it incapable of producing more electricity. That is, integrative energy which cannot be restored when electricity runs out. What depletes it then, is not the generation of electricity, but entropy. Likewise, the "body battery" cannot be perpetually "recharged" by oxygen, food, and drink.

The energy in question, then, is the *fundamental* one of two which integrate the molecular structures of the electromagnet's battery's chemicals. This is all quite scientific. It is the *analogy* that does not hold. The biochemicals in the cells and fluids of a naturally dying, hence still living, person, unlike those in a dying battery, are the same as they always were. What does change at this point, and prior to it as the individual grows old, occurs, of course, at a higher level of organization. When we speak of life, we speak also of cellular organization and, in the case of humans, tissue and organ organization above that, with distribution of substances in fluids and of fluids in organs. What changes is cell replacement, tissue regeneration, and metabolic energy; all are less. The distributional factors are consequences of this. And the simple fact is, "science" can say nothing whatever about an analog of the battery's molecule-binding energy that pertains to the biological level of cell, tissue, organic, and metabolic integration. There is no "heart-kidney-liver-lung-spleen-brain-etc. molecule." Western science leaves off at the inanimate level of chemicals, as far as energy is concerned.

Because rubber is an organic material, it serves better than battery fluid to illustrate the hole in Western science which bio-energy fills. A strip of rubber wound to spin the prop of a model airplane stores energy. It serves the purpose of a chemical battery, but stores and yields far more energy by weight. Its unwinding energy is transferred to the prop shaft to which it is connected. Through initial use, its length when not under tension is extended and its cross section decreased. As a result, its torque (turning force) decreases, but the number of times it turns increases, so the amounts of energy it can absorb and yield remain the same. Structural change of form, then, has nothing to do with what happens after this breaking-in process. Nor does biochemical structure. What happens is that through use it becomes less and less capable of absorbing and yielding energy. The chemically organic battery runs down.

In Western scientific terms, change associated with this loss of capacity may be described in terms of changes in the "tissue" structure of the rubber strip. But this only reinforces the implication that an integrative form of energy *operating above the level of biochemical structure* must have been present in a definite amount and been decreased, mainly or entirely during use, by entropy. Similarly, at a level of complexity far higher than in this "half alive" (organic but inanimate) example, at the start of life there is bioenergy in a definite amount, which is eventually exhausted by entropy via the living process.

The integrative energies fundamental to the continued potential of the electrochemical battery, the rubber strip, and the human organism are all recognized as forms of chi from the Chinese scientific perspective. It is *biological* chi, i.e., chi exclusive to living individuals, that is unknown to Western science.

(2) A Third (Unknown) Factor With the exception of unnatural death due to intervening causes, proposition 2, that altered biochemistry and exhaustion of bioenergy are effects of a third factor, is defective in the way opposite to that of proposition 1. It is not too little, but too much—logically redundant. It violates the rule of thought economy, Occam's razor, unnecessarily proposing a third variable where two are explanatorily sufficient. We can explain dying in terms of biochemical substance and bioenergy, understanding entropy always to be operative.

(3) *The Chinese Scientific Proposition* Before death and the distinctive acidity of the corpse, there is a "running out" of bioenergy of a type unknown to Western science. There is no way of escaping this implication. Western scientists can point at and describe in unparalleled detail a decline in metabolic energy and regenerative capacity (and their effects, e.g., fluid deficiency, arteriosclerosis, osteoporosis), but as soon as they state or suggest these are the *causes* of natural dying (and they may, as they have no other option), they are refusing to answer the question at hand: How does a human die of *natural* causes? The only logical answer is: The bioenergy runs out.

But let us take a closer look at this bioenergy. Actually, we have been speaking of two kinds. Again, the electromagnet analogy is useful. We proceeded from a "hair-on-my-head" organizing field, like the iron filings–patterning EM field, to a fundamental lifetime energy, like the nonrechargeable energy binding molecules in the battery's chemicals. Here we focus on the latter. Just as the electromagnet cannot have a field without a coil and integral chemicals in its battery, the human body cannot have a field without cellular, tissue, and organic substance and structure, and basic bioenergy that is attached to, and assumedly integrates, that substance and structure. And, like the electromagnet's nonrechargeable binding energy, that basic bioenergy is in a *potential* state as far as material "sensing" or metering devices are concerned. Only that part of the energy lost through entropy during a given period could be detected in this way—assumedly, as heat.

It is important to understand that this basic bioenergy is not electromagnetic, or, when doing its vital job, caloric. If it were, the field would decline from birth, or we would live only as long as food is available. In turn, we have no term for it. Indeed, we would not even know how to go about conducting laboratory experiments to determine its nature—if that were possible or ethical. It is "something" Western science is conceptually and technologically unequipped to deal with—and certainly this has much to do with its illogical treatment of the basic question we have asked, and its attempt to reduce chi to mere electromagnetism and biochemical effect. The Chinese scientific term for this basic bioenergy is *yuan chi*, "original" chi (see fig. 1-4: Chi Chart). It is called original because it is (must be) present at the beginning of life, for it is plainly indispensable to living.

Now that I have drawn a sharp line, I add that—as the electromagnet analogy suggests—this original chi is not EM energy as we know it, but is like EM energy and may be a kind of EM energy that we don't yet know. As for formative chi, discussed below, of course it is electromagnetic, though it has some properties which cannot be accounted for in such terms.

To respect Western science's criterion of measurability (but not its terms or its means of measuring), we can say that original chi is measurable, but not at any "one time." Its amount is directly proportionate to the amount of energy metabolically and formatively processed by an individual in a lifetime ended by natural death, for this is the energetic flow it potentiates, and which ceases when it runs out.

Original chi can also be "gauged" at a given time, as the basic element in the "force qualities" expertly perceived by the pulse-feeling fingertips of a Chinese physician. Indeed, a Chinese physician of highest order can tell in this way if a person will die naturally within a week to a month, before there might be any clinical signs of such an event. What he senses is a depletion of this chi. Of the numerous force qualities of the pulse, the one in question is *shen*, a term which is usually, and somewhat misleadingly, translated as *spirit* (see fig. 1-5, p. 24), but which in this context could be translated as "vital coherency and rhythmicity." Here, actualized original chi is intimately intermixed with metabolic energies, but remains the salient aspect. Of course, Western science cannot be brought to bear on such a matter, because it has never developed a sense of qualities, nor the perceptiveness or aesthetic sensitivity of those who practice

Figure 1-4: Chi Chart

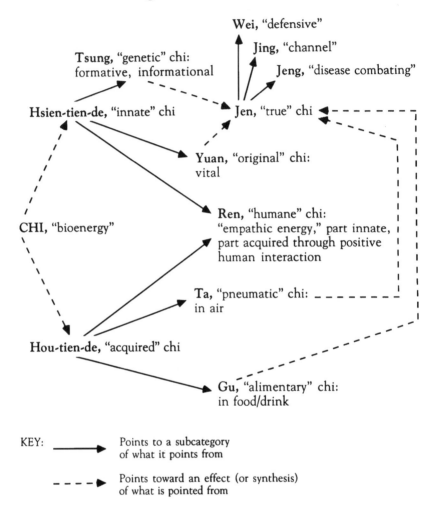

KEY:

⟶   Points to a subcategory of what it points from

— — ▶   Points toward an effect (or synthesis) of what is pointed from

Definitions are given following the colon(:).

Translational glosses are given in quotes (" ").

it.[19] And if it were to produce a sensing device adequate to testing such Chinese theory, it would have produced a human being—a business rightly reserved for mothers and fathers.[20]

Manifestations of Chi What has been explained so far may suggest that entropy (*guei*) is the opposite of chi. Actually entropy opposes organic substance as much as it does bioenergy. This introduces yet another meaning of chi, a cosmological one often confused with the bioenergetic chi of chi gong, acupuncture, and herbal medicine. Like the term for original chi, this one is romanized as *yuan chi*, but the romanization is of homonyms. The literal sense of this *yuan* is "primal." Primal chi is hyperenergy matter—what "remains" when the polarity between energy and matter is neutralized by entropy, and what "exists" before polarization (see fig. 1-5). This primal cosmological extreme is what the *tai ji* diagram (fig. 1-1) represents: the universe at the extreme "point" of change (*ji*) in its evolutive-devolutive cycle, or "The Changer" itself. It is at this "level" that *guei*/entropy has an opposite, and it is not chi, but *shen* (spirit). *Shen* is the polarizing, energizing and materializing force; *guei* is the depolarizing, deenergizing and dematerializing force (see fig. 1-5).

The prephilosophical Greeks saw it the same way. Their Eros equals *shen* and their Thanatos equals *guei*. (Eros, in the primary sense meaning "love," like love is an integrating force; Thanatos, in the primary sense meaning "death," like death is a disintegrating force.) But the Chinese Taoists took logical comprehension one step further, recognizing that there must be a factor of some degree of independence which was/is responsible for the integrativeness or disintegrativeness of a cycle—the macrocosmological correlate of what we have been examining. This ultimate causal factor is called either *tai-ji* or Tao (pronounced Dow). *Tai-ji* emphasizes the inchoate dynamics of *shen* and *guei*. Tao emphasizes the way change proceeds and its obligatory power.

Figure 1-5: The Cosmological Context of Chi (Bioenergy)

Tao or *Tai-Ji*:
"the way" or "the extreme point of change"; "the changer."

Thanatos	Eros
Guei, entropy,	*Shen*, spirit,
The depolarizing, disintegrating force	The polarizing integrating force
(deenergizing and dematerializing).	(energizing and materializing).

Yuan* Chi, cosmic chi,
The basic "stuff" of the universe,
hyper-energy-matter.

Depolarized cosmic chi:
nothing, emptiness,
oblivion

Fully polarized cosmic chi:
The cosmos in full bloom,
cosmic Eden

Nearly full to nearly empty
Shui, substance
Ti, structure

Nearly full to nearly empty
Chi, integrating
formative energy

Yin

Yang

Hsüeh, organic matter   Chi, bioenergy

KEY: ⟶   Points to an aspect of what it is pointing from

⟹   Points to what it transforms

- - -▶   Points to what it transforms into, or toward

*Literally "primal." A romanization of a Chinese character other than the *yuan*, "original," on the Chi Chart (fig. 1-4).

Shen and *guei* are the fundamental forces and as such do not require much attention here. They are always operative, so, once understood, can be ignored, except insofar as our own activities align with one or the other. It is at the level of the energetic-material cosmos (cosmos means "organization") that we directly participate and exert influences. At this level, cosmological chi is differentiated into chi (as energy) on the *yang* side, and *hsüeh*, what we call matter (*ti*, "structure," or *shui*, literally "water" or substance), on the *yin* side.

When the matter is organized and incorporated in living individuals, it is called *hsüeh*. Biochemical substances are structurally deep components of *hsüeh* discovered by Western scientists. In the Chinese conception, *hsüeh* can be infinitely broken down into components of components, but the smallest operative concept is the cell, *hsi-bao*. The opposite of chi in the basic sense of this book, then, is *hsüeh*. This is where figure 1-5 ends and the Chi Chart (fig. 1-4) begins, with chi (at the far left) distinguished from *hsüeh*, as "bio-energy." Chi gives form and movement to *hsüeh*, and *hsüeh* gives chi a place "to be-at." Neither can exist without the other. Without chi, *hsüeh* decomposes, to become inorganic. Without *hsüeh*, chi is not present. Each helps the other to defeat (or forestall) entropy/*guei*. In Judeo-Christian terms, chi is the "breath of God" and *hsüeh* is the "clay" (as used in the story of creation in Genesis).

When genuine masters of chi gong and Chinese medicine speak of chi in the environment, then, they are referring to neither innate nor cosmological chi; it is not a channelled force in the *Star Wars* sense. There is, however, knowledge of potentiating interactions between the body (including its chi) and the local environment, (including its chi), which are too numerous to discuss here. Such knowledge is used both in developing *gong fu* (special abilities) and in minimizing expenditure of energy.

An example of developing gong-fu is the practice of gruelling martial arts exercises performed when the sun is at its peak to challenge maximally the *yang* energies of the practitioner against the "great *yang*" of the sun. (*Don't try this on your own*; initiates must be professionally supervised or they may become severely ill!) Such ideas originate and are fully apprehended through intuitive perception and spirit. They have virtually nothing to do with science as we know it.

It is in that sense that those possessed of *gong fu* may be said to be in touch with, in harmony with, or empowered by chi in the (nonhuman) environment, i.e., chi other than the energy metabolically absorbed from air, drink, and food. They have developed special capacities in part by interacting intimately and knowledgeably with what we now tend to mean by "nature." There is also an empowering human chi which *is* like the *Star Wars* force, which we will discuss soon.

We now understand that innate chi and *hsüeh* are on an equal par; there is no spiritual (or material) bias. It is just that in the biological process of change in a lifetime, it is the interplay between original chi and entropy/*guei* that is causally primary—unless extraordinary circumstances intervene. For example, a person may be starved, bled, or sweated to death. In such instances, loss of *hsueh* is the initial cause of dying. The original chi lacks "place to be-at," and so "runs out" prior to natural term. As it does so, the organizational field recedes, like a fountain whose source has dried up, and disorganization at all structural levels ensues, from "top" (metabolism) through death to "bottom" (chemical structure).

Similarly, as a person grows old the original chi declines, so does metabolism. As a result fluids become less nutritive and less in volume and distribution, and tissues harden. The organizational field then weakens and recedes, and there is less formative-regenerative capacity (of this, more in a moment). That Chinese medicine can prolong life, that is, vitality and well-being, and in this sense slow the aging process, is due to its understanding of the affinities of certain herbs to original chi and its immediate energetic sphere of actualization. (Actually, the combinations and relative proportions of these herbs is as important as the herbs themselves.) Chi gong may be used supportively, to minimize expenditure of original chi and maximize circulation and metabolism.

Innate Chi The difference and relation between original chi and formative chi is indicated by the electromagnet analogy. The energy in the electromagnetic field is a potential of the energy in the battery (to which original chi is analogous) and of the copper coil (to which the energetic conduits of the living body are analogous). The formative pattern that iron filings move through to assume the shape of the EM field is like the formative pattern that fetal cells move through to assume a human shape. The inconsistency in this analogy points at the inanimate/animate difference. In an electromagnet the coil is already present before there is an organizational field, but in the case of fetal development, the energetic conduits themselves are a product of the developmental process. It follows from this that the formative chi in a fetally developing organism, unlike the EM organizational field of an electromagnet, is not a mere product of a basic energy and its conduits. Rather, it has an existence of its own, and it must be present before development can occur.

Of course, there is some scientific evidence to this effect. Kirlian electrophotographs of living organisms from which parts have been amputated, show the shape of the amputated part. That is, when *some* of the biochemical (and cell and tissue, and if it is a complex organism, organ) substance is present, *all* of the formative EM field is present. (Nevertheless when too much substance is lost, so is the field.)

It may seem we have jumped to conclusions, until the holes in Western science's explanations of fetal development are pointed out. "Science" recognizes that there must be instructions for fetal development (and cell replacement of correct kind in correct place in the tissue regenerating process), and it describes this process in terms of biochemical cell composition, cell production, cell travel, and tissue and organ formation with a detail and precision that Chinese medicine could not approach. But it does not (and could not) *explain* the phenomenon. It only promises to, given the time and money for more research. If it ever does, it will no longer be Western science, because it would have to have borrowed or independently created the concept of chi, and to do so would fundamentally alter our scientific paradigm. Indeed, in an extraordinary book, *A New Science of Life*,[21] Dr. Rupert Sheldrake, an English biologist, quite independently of Chinese science, demonstrates on the basis of fascinating biological evidence that there must be formative fields which are present continually through the generations.

Sheldrake rightly does not define these fields in scientific—i.e., electromagnetic or biochemical—terms. From the Chinese scientific perspective, this is too metaphysical a conceptualization. Formative chi in living context does have an EM aspect, but the point is rightly made that mainstream modern biology, at least, does not (but should) contain such a variable. (As Sheldrake observes, the Western biological notion of a formative field of some kind is not new; rather, it has never been developed, nor have its implications been fully explored. It has been cast aside by mainstream biology.)

To propose, in mainstream Western biological terms, that biochemical substances in cells and a small number of fetal cells in a certain, primitive, symmetrical aggregation incorporate all the variables required for individual development is like saying that if a section of the EM coil is removed, there will still be a field, and that the field will cause *copper* filings in its vicinity to form the missing part of the coil. No degree of complexity, viewed as information, in the chemical structures of the battery could relieve this proposition of absurdity.

But that is essentially what mainstream biology proposes: genetic biochemical substances in fetal cells are a "code" which not only contains the information, but, somehow, brings about the complex, sequenced, differentiating action, including cell travel, required for a spherical organization of identical cells to grow into a human form. This is tantamount to saying that a ball bearing made of steel alloy X when heated to the melting point will assume the form of a human-oid figurine, every time, and that the information and the formative energies or forces for this transformation are the molecular structure of alloy X. What's more, a ball bearing made of steel alloy Y will assume the form of, say, an arthropoid (spider-like) figurine, every time, exclusively by virtue of the molecular structure of alloy Y.

Certainly, biochemical and EM processes are essential to the formation of a fetus, and to the regeneration of tissue; but to propose that such phenomena are *caused* in their entirety by biochemical substances—most of which, to boot, are the *effects* of such processes—is quite absurd, especially when we can make Kirlian electrophotographs of the "missing" variable! Rather, it makes good sense to understand that what genetic scientists call "genetic infor-mation" is not that, but chemical substances that are responsive to the genetically informative and *formation-enabling* energy field, some-what in the way that iron filings are responsive to an EM field. Western science has mistaken the lock for the key!

The kind of chi which forms living organic matter, then, is present at conception with the original chi. With descriptive accu-racy, it is called *tsung* chi (literally, kind-chi): genetic, or ancestral, chi (see fig. 1-4). It is what formatively causes fetal development and tissue regeneration later in life according to kind (e.g., human, male or female, fibrocartilaginous cell, and specific ancestry).

Hsien-tien-de chi (see fig. 1-4) is simply a term which denotes both original chi and genetic chi. It means "innate" chi, given at conception. Literally translated, *hsien-tien* means "prior nature," and so implies the theory of innate chi. It is associated primarily with the kidneys, secondarily with the heart (the two original fetal organs, or *orbs*, i.e., organs and functions[22]).

It is worth pointing out that the manipulation of genetic biochemical substances in DNA experiments to produce unprecedented (and from a Chinese medical, ecological, or human intuitive position, monstrous) life-forms, does not prove that such biochemical structures are all that is essential to life. Rather, if logic is allowed to illuminate the matter fully, such laboratory deformations of the generative and developmental vital process imply that when genetic matter is displaced, so is genetic chi.

Acquired Chi We turn now from innate kinds of chi to "acquired" chi, that is, chi which enters the living organism in the process of living. This kind of bioenergy is the same as the one recognized by "science," and links innate chi to the remaining kinds of chi (those not recognized by "science") on the Chi Chart (fig. 1-4). The Chinese term *hou-tien-de*, acquired chi, or that "of latter nature," contrasts with *hsien-tien-de*, chi "of prior nature." If innate chi is responsible for the formation and continued integrity of the organism, acquired chi is the quintessence of the organism's vital fuel. The first acquired chi received in a lifetime is extracted, by energy provided from the actualization of original chi, from the water (amniotic fluid) surrounding the fetus and the nutritive organic matter which enters through the umbilical cord. Note that without positing original chi, that is, a given energy, there is no way to account for initial metabolism of oxygen and food. (To explain this primary energy as the mother's is to ignore *her* developmental growth and the innate chi actualizations gestation implies.)

The chi extracted from the amniotic fluid is a close correlate of that metabolic catalyst we call oxygen. It is called *ta* chi (pneumatic chi, see fig. 1-4)—literally, great chi, referring to the greatest sector of our natural environment, the atmosphere. This chi is extracted at first from the atmosphere by the mother's lung orb (orb meaning organ and function) and via the kidney orb enters the "atmosphere" surrounding the fetus, to be extracted by the fetus through proto lung orbs. After birth, the human's own lung orb performs this function; hence the lungs are among the orbs qualified as "of latter nature."

The conversion of ingested food substance into bioenergy, *gu* chi, or alimentary chi (see fig. 1-4), requires catalysis by *ta*, pneumatic chi. In Chinese theory, two processes are involved. One is that via the bloodstream from the lung orb pneumatic chi joins digested food in the large-intestine orb to produce the alimentary chi (and its substantial substratum) which nourishes all orbs via the bloodstream. The other is that the kidneys, the "watery" orb, attract and absorb pneumatic chi directly from the lung orb to produce a general metabolism-energizing bioenergy which is likened to rising steam or vapor (the semantically basic meaning of the word *chi*).

Actually, according to Chinese theory there is a little more to pneumatic chi than "oxygen" (i.e., a catalyzing substance), but there is no great difference here with Western biochemistry. Pneumatic chi is understood to contain an energy which potentially is heat, coming from the sun and all other radiating celestial bodies. It is not called chi, but *yang*. Its potential is realized when it enters the water (kidney orb) of the body, and the result is chi in the sense of steam, or vapor, a warmth and uprising fluid without which the organs (the anatomical substrates of orbs) could not function. In Western terms this warmth is caloric energy released when oxygen inhaled is exchanged by carbon dioxide exhaled. The "physiology" is different, but both cultures are talking about heat.

Now, at last, we can understand the *jen* chi, true chi, to which those possessed of *gong fu* centrally refer when they speak of their special abilities. *Jen* means "true," and truth in the Chinese scientific understanding is the conceptual key. What is true is what is fully accounted for. What is true is real in the sense "maximally present," and what is maximally present is a focal function, or functional nexus, of everything essentially related to it. In short, *jen* implies a complex and whole entity, holistically conceptualized and understood, which, because it is complex and whole, is of maximum presence and therefore maximum power. Accordingly, *jen* chi is indicated on the Chi Chart (fig. 1-4) as the nexus, or synthesis, of the two types of innate chi and of the two types of acquired chi. We could say that "true chi" is the synthesis and quintessence of all the other kinds of chi we have discussed.

It is impractical to describe all the essential relationships among chis (not to mention essential substances) that form the essence of true chi, but a selective review may further clarify the matter. Without original chi, there is disintegration and vital arhythmia of the organism. Without acquired and formative chi, there is no actualization of original chi. Without genetic chi, there is no formation or regeneration of the organism. Without acquired and original chi, there is no metabolism. So, without *jen* chi, there is no life. It is important to understand that *jen* chi is not merely a catchall term. Each chi interacts with and *changes* the others. *Jen* chi is not X-chi plus Y-chi, but the complex reality of these interactions. Only in *jen* chi do we have a realistic, as opposed to analytically rigorous, concept.

Chi gong, or exercises of the chi, can now be understood. For a central example, there is the image of replenishing, raising, and circulating chi concentrated below the navel. What is being replenished is the actualizing potential of the original chi and the formative potential of the genetic chi, mainly via correct breathing and correct imaging, respectively. The raising is of both the vapor and the (electromagnetic) genetic chi, and the circulating is of the true chi. It is easy to understand why the area below the navel is the focal starting point, and why it and chi gong are associated with regeneration and the fetus. Likewise, the importance of correct breathing is directly related to the vital rhythmic contribution of original chi and its latter-natural correlate, breathing.

Now we are going to enter a new, external, dimension of chi and chi gong, and in doing so we will begin to think less in terms of kinds of energy and more in terms of waves and vibrations. Of course, these are only two aspects of the same thing. These waves and vibrations constitute the chi atmosphere that is generated by human beings.

The interface between the chi of the organism and this "atmosphere" is *wei* chi (or defensive chi, see fig. 1-4), which is, in fact, thoroughly intermixed with genetic chi to leave the impression of an aura in Kirlian photographs, and to activate electromagnetic sensing devices. Defensive chi is not another kind of chi, but an aspect of the true chi that surrounds the visible palpable body. Its internal counterpart is *jeng* chi, the bioenergy which homeostatically combats disease (see fig. 1-4). "Between" them is *jing* chi, true chi conducted along *jing*, the channels or pathways, to which we have strategic access using acupuncture points, which are not "points" in a Cartesian sense, but physiologically and medically strategic nexuses of true chi.

In Chinese medical understanding, defensive chi, like a force-field in Western imagery, actually repels pathogens (disease-causing energies and microorganisms), as makes perfectly good common and scientific sense. Chi gong masters, apparently able to withstand incursions of physical objects which would maim or kill normal people, have expanded this concept when they attribute such capacities to chi (see the photographs of hard chi in the Introduction). On the basis of my own martial arts experience, I do believe that defensive chi contributes to the integrity of stressed flesh, but I would guess that physical cultivation in the standard sense, coupled with special know-how, is essential to such demonstrations, some of which are convincing and some not.

A more important aspect of external chi is a far more subtle and common interaction than the one just exemplified. It is a phenomenon of waves and vibrations, which, I believe, is sometimes unintentionally misrepresented by Chinese individuals as a force directly exerted on the physical constitution of inanimate objects, plants, animals, or people. At the apex of such interactions is the last of the chis on the Chi Chart (fig. 1-4): *ren* chi, humane chi, in the sense "humane and human." The character *Jen* includes the character for human being. In Chinese, "humane" presupposes healthy human nature and interaction, as a sufficient basis. No divine or supernatural influence is involved.

Ren chi is the healthy and directly life-promoting type of external chi, that is, of chi that functions between or among individuals. It is rooted in and comes from psychologically and socially healthy individuals. We could say that it is true chi plus one's "mind and heart." It embodies the intentions, will, spiritual attention, attitudes, and emotions of such an individual at a given moment and as a continuing influence in the human chi atmosphere. This space does not permit an attempt to define those additional variables. Suffice it to say that some are forms of chi, and some are aspects of (rather than additions to) true chi, and that the complex net product is in part electromagnetic, sound, and heat energy. But in greater part it is waves or vibrations which laboratory devices cannot sense, but sensitive human beings can. More importantly, all humans can and do respond to it. Given the logical conclusions defining true chi, it is reasonable to posit such extremely subtle influences and human responsive capacity. Instead of logic, then, here are some examples which might be familiar.

People in the sixties, like me, spoke of "good vibrations," and their antithesis, "bad vibrations." The positive concept was quickly debased by imitation and popular music, but it originally referred to a spiritual-sensory experience, honestly and aptly described. Good vibrations, I say, are interactions between the humane chis emitted by human beings.

According to Chinese *shang-yi*, "higher medicine," humane chi can be cultivated, primarily through education that is both intellectual and emotional, and is rooted in chi gong and physical exercise. To characterize such education briefly, it is based on love of other human beings and all other forms of life. It is believed that such self-cultivation imbues humane chi with special potency, namely, to influence others in such positive direction. An example within the medical sphere as we usually think of it is healing which involves no more than personal presence, healing intention and, usually, touching. By no means is this a capacity exclusive to healers. It is just that they can do it most widely. Close relatives and spouses are especially able to do it, and do so naturally.

The scientific aspect of it is that there is an interaction between the chis of two or more human beings, as the causal, or effective, reality, and that this feeds back all the way to the internal, organic level.

If there is such external chi, it stands to reason that interpersonal chi may take other forms, i.e., have different vibrations with different effects, from the above. We know that fluorescent lights scramble some people's brain waves—a phenomenon of wave interference—and that colors powerfully influence moods and even the degree to which strength is exerted. Infrasound, also at the long-waved, subtle end of the spectrum, may sap energy. It is realistically conceivable, therefore, that it is possible for some people to emanate chi which influences other people's thoughts, levels of awareness, direction of attention, and physical capacities. The potential here for extraordinary demonstrations, or exercises of external chi, is considerable (as will be shown in chapters 7 and 9). At the luminous side is the potential to humanely transform and heal, even at a distance. At the dark side is what we call black magic or Satanism, which thrives in all cultures in one form or another, when culture in the genuine sense of systematized humane influences, and its infrastructure, humane political and economic institutions, have degenerated. Between these poles and well within the luminous sector are demonstrations of special external chi capacities, be they fully genuine or partaking of the techniques of stage magic.

If true chi is the "chi of chis" in the internal sphere, humane chi is the equivalent in the external one. It is the aura of genuine culture and civilization, the warm and gentle atmosphere which human beings at their best emanate by way of completing our potential to self-actualize as members of our species. In theory and in reputable experience, the emanation of humane chi from individuals has a mutually amplifying, synergically energizing effect, quite apparent, for example, in certain types (and there are many) of group dancing. Perhaps more focused attention to this and related ideas will be conducive to more spiritual-sensory contact with and generation of the reality they conceptualize. All regenerations and improvements of culture and its implementing institutions begin with what may be called aligned and mutually magnifying positive human impulses.

As with the holistic nature of truth, ultimately the health of the extrahuman sphere is also essential to the presence of humane chi, and, reciprocally, humane chi and its infrastructures are essential to the health of our environment. The Satanic, proentropic slaughter of the forests which is the emblem and core of our current destruction, deprives us of air, the atmosphere of the soul. (My choice of words is not deliberate but inevitable: the *guei*, faithfully translated as "entropy," above, is the same word which, in human context, means "ill-intentioned anti-human-being.") As our natural place degenerates, so does the bioenergetic potential of any form of chi gong. Reciprocally, revival of our ecosphere would make chi gong a special aspect of our joy in being alive and human.

Notes

1. For a more thorough explanation see: Bruce Holbrook, *The Stone Monkey: An Alternative Chinese-Scientific Reality* (New York: William Morrow, 1981), 227–230; and Manfred Porkert, *The Theoretical Foundations of Chinese Medicine: Systems of Correspondence* (Cambridge, Mass.: M.I.T. Press, 1974).

2. Barbara Brown, in her research into biofeedback, developed many insights that would be shared by chi gong masters, for instance: (a) humans have innate biological awareness of their physical state, down to the level of the single cell; (b) humans can control the direction and flow of nerve impulses throughout the body; (c) the mind can intervene in and direct any physiologic function; (d) the mind controls the physical

activity of the brain; (*e*) the highest order intellectual capacities reside in what we call the unconscious. Barbara Brown, *Supermind* (New York: Harper and Row, 1979).

3. A *shih* is a traditional Chinese savant who "has achieved full florescence as a human being tutored in and practicing taxing forms of intellectual, emotional, and physical self-cultivation" (Holbrook, *The Stone Monkey*, 11). *Shih-fu* is the title for a savant, given by an apprentice.

4. Holbrook, *The Stone Monkey*, 229.

5. Cyrus Lee, "Personal Reflections on Qigong," *Psi Research*, March 1984, 86. The quote was translated by Dr. Lee from Master Guo's book *A New Methodology of Qigong Applied in Cancer Treatment* (Shanghai: The Scientific Press, 1981), 1.

6. Xu Hong-zhang and Zhao Yong-jie, "An Approach to Psi Radiation Signals," *Psi Research*, Dec. 1982, 17.

7. *Jing* chi is a compound of vital quintessence (*jing*) and vital energy (chi); it is not a kind of chi. Also understood as meridian chi (*jing luo zhi* chi) whose circulation along the meridians in the body can be directed.

8. I. Veith, trans., *The Yellow Emperor's Classic of Internal Medicine*, 2d ed. (Berkeley: Univ. of California Press, 1972).

9. David Eisenberg precedes his account of personally witnessed extraordinary experiences by pointing out, "Qi Gong masters claim to control their Qi absolutely, directing it through any portion of their body at will in order to perform seemingly superhuman feats." David Eisenberg, *Encounters with Qi: Exploring Chinese Medicine* (New York: Penguin, 1987), 48.

10. An infrasonic wave has a frequency below sixteen hertz and is inaudible to humans. One characteristic of infrasound is that it decays very little while traveling through the air and therefore can travel many miles.

11. Xie Huan-zhang, *The Scientific Basis of Chi Gong* (Beijing: Beijing Institute of Technology, 1985).

12. Cf., R. Becker and G. Selden, *The Body Electric: Electromagnetism and the Foundation of Life* (New York: William Morrow, 1985).

13. As published in *Nature* Magazine (Shanghai: Vol 1 No 1, 1981), p. 43.

14. ibid. p. 44.

15. Robin Baker, in *New Scientist* 87 (1980): 844–46.

16. Paul Dong, in manuscript of "Chi Gong Instructions."

17. The well-known image of a yogi lying on a bed of spikes allies the Indian concept of prana, activated by yoga, to the Chinese chi, activated by chi gong.

18. Typically, the bone cells contain less calcium, but this is not known to be a cause of death, and even if it were, it is not predictable from biochemical cell structure. Other features of the typical aged body pertain to levels of organization higher than the

biochemical one, some of which may be partially described in biochemical terms, e.g., fluid composition, but none of these are predictive causes of death or predictable from biochemical cell structure.

19. To the reader interested in understanding the basic difference between Western and Chinese science and medicine and the Chinese science of qualities, I highly recommend: Manfred Porkert, *Chinese Medicine: Its History, Philosophy, and Practice, and Why It May One Day Dominate the Medicine of the West* (New York: William Morrow, 1988).

20. This is not to imply that pulse-force qualities do not register distinct patterns on such devices or that they do not have great clinical utility. Michael Broffman, C.A., of San Anselmo, Ca., an accomplished, traditionally trained healer, offers pulse imagery using such a device. The point is that fully sensitive diagnosis requires a direct, human-to-human relationship.

21. Rupert Sheldrake, *A New Science of Life* (Los Angeles: Tarcher, 1981).

22. For an explanation of organs in Western biology and orbs, which are at once anatomical and functional entities, see: Manfred Porkert, *The Theoretical Foundations of Chinese Medicine.*

2

Healing and Health Through Chi Gong

Without chi there is no Chinese Medicine.

—Professor Ren Ying-qin[1]

China, with a huge population of a billion people, lacks both doctors and medicine. Until quite recently all hospitals and clinics were run by the government. Patients had to line up for many hours to see a doctor. In recent years, more private doctors have become available, but their fees are often too high. In general, access to health care can be very difficult. Chi gong offers an alternative. For many conditions Chinese learn chi gong for self-treatment or seek external chi therapy without consulting either a doctor of Western medicine or a doctor of traditional Chinese medicine. We advise against this practice without prior consultation with a licensed medical doctor.

The use of external chi in the treatment of many diseases has become widely accepted in China. External chi therapy, one of the methods of chi gong health practice, requires neither medication or injection, nor any physical contact with the patient. Usually the chi is released from between two inches to a foot away from the body, and the treatment may take three to thirty minutes. Some patients are cured with one treatment, but more often it takes three daily

39

treatments to obtain results. This therapy is at present very popular in China; at least ten million treatments are given yearly. For instance, Dr. Zhao Kuang of the Xi Wang Hospital of Traditional Chinese Medicine gives about two thousand treatments annually. It is estimated that over a thousand chi gong masters in China have mastered the skill.

The essence of external chi therapy is the passage of energy from the chi gong master to the patient, fortifying the patient's own ability to fight disease. It may be likened to the recharging of a rundown car battery. According to traditional Chinese medicine, a person becomes ill when chi and blood are not circulating well and therefore the yin and yang are out of balance. Either acupuncture or the application of external chi or both can improve directly the circulation of life energy and blood and thus right the imbalance between yin and yang.

Despite the fact that the American public is familiar only with Western medical and technological knowledge, and despite the prevailing scepticism about natural and traditional medical practices in general, Paul Dong's wife encouraged him to write about his own experiences, telling him, "Since you are of great help to our whole family, you should write about the beautiful happenings under the moonlight."

"Beautiful happenings under the moonlight" refers to the health-care instruction or treatment that Dong gives his wife and children, usually when there is moonlight, or three days before and after the full moon. Chi gong, in its long history, has developed many legends, and one holds that the best results both in training and therapy can be obtained during the three days before and after the full moon. In chi gong terminology, "full moon and summer" indicates the best time for exercise. In summer it is warm and one can practice in the field, by the riverside or by a lake, under a tree or in a meadow. The gravitational pull of the moon, just as it causes the tides of the ocean, exerts an influence on the practice of chi gong and how it affects the body.

The following is an example of Dong's treatments:

On October 7, 1987, it was full moon. Since five o'clock in the afternoon, my wife had complained of a painful lump in the chest, experiencing a painful area as large as a fist. She was in bed, feeling a heavy load pressing her down. She had no appetite for food or drink. When the moon came out at about 7 P.M., she asked me to treat her with chi gong. I put out my hand and sent my external chi from the *lao-gong* point in my palm and left it in the two-inch area of pain for three minutes. The lump dissolved and her pain left. But a few moments later she was again groaning in pain. I knew that I had to repeat the treatment for a longer time. It again took about three minutes for the lump to disappear. After seven minutes my wife told me that she felt as if a stream of hot gas, or steam, spiraled down from her chest to her navel. After ten minutes she felt warm all over and only then did I stop the release of my chi. The painful lump had vanished and when I asked her how she was feeling, she answered that she felt fine all over, clearer in the head, with a sense of euphoria.

Apart from practicing healing on his family, Dong also helps his students during chi gong class. He has been teaching chi gong since 1985, but has been able to release external chi only since the beginning of 1987. His healing can alleviate pain, as well as colds, stuffed noses, dizziness, back and head aches, sleeplessness, high blood pressure, and some chronic conditions.[2] At this time results are about 50 percent positive, and he knows that the strength of his external chi may increase by 10 to 15 percent annually, depending on how much he practices daily.

According to the best available Chinese statistics the overall efficacy rate of external chi treatment is 50 percent, while for those patients who practice chi gong themselves the rate may go up to approximately 70 percent. If the patient can be induced to spend more than one hour daily in chi gong practice, the individual's improvement or cure rate can be much higher (see also chapters 4 and 5).

For the Chinese, and many others in the East, the activation of life energy is of essence to good health and longevity. For Americans, the therapeutic practice of chi gong would pose many problems. For instance, Western medicine would not even begin to consider the influence of the moon in either understanding illness or practicing healing. Then, most Western medical practice, except for "talk therapy," requires touching the patient. Body/mind communication as the path to self-healing is readily accepted by many Eastern cultures, but the Western mindset regarding this ancient way of healing is radically different.

The Split Between Body and Mind in Conventional Western Science

The sharp difference in how the East and the West experience the world originated relatively recently. The Western Judeo-Christian and the Chinese Taoist-Confucian worldviews probably began to differ radically some two thousand years ago.[3] However, even as late as the Middle Ages the process of healing was not experienced differently by men and women the world over. It was not until the seventeenth century and Descartes, the first modern philosopher, that Western thinking has come to accept a split between mind and matter, never thought of before and not recognized in Chinese thinking.

Descartes formulated parallel realms: *matter* that can be measured (because, for one, it is divisible and occupies space) and *mind* that cannot be scientifically studied (because it is indivisible and does not occupy space). His aim was to avoid the moral and political conflicts of his day. As a scientist he wanted to pursue the new insights into the relations between humans and their universe, while as a Roman Catholic philosopher he feared the Inquisition of the church. After all, at age twenty-six he had learned that the church, which had held to the traditional and erroneous view that the sun revolves around the earth, had punished Galileo for proving the opposite.

The most regrettable consequence of Descartes' separation of mind and matter was that the human being, heretofore a union of body and soul, also came to be seen as consisting of two separable and distinct substances. Even though each of us experiences his or her self as one, Descartes proposed that only the body, as part of the physical universe, could be studied scientifically. Since mind (or the soul) is connected to god and cannot be measured, Descartes decided it should not be studied or interfered with by science. He thought himself to have been clever, because this dualism would satisfy the Roman Catholic Church, which claimed to represent divine reality and thus had control over human truth. To get around the church's strictures, Descartes proposed that science be left alone to develop its view of matter, while theology would retain its jurisdiction over mind. But this "Cartesian compromise" was flawed from the beginning, because, as we now know, the *transactions* between mind/body cannot be accepted without either destroying the mechanism of science or the independence of mind. In 1669, within twenty years of Descartes' death, the Inquisition placed some of his works on the index of books forbidden to be read by Catholics. However, his intellectual compromise continued on as the solution to many philosophical problems. The modern scientific worldview from its beginning was under the influence of Descartes' dualism, and this distortion in our thinking has only recently begun to lessen.[4]

In the last two hundred years, practitioners of Western science and technology have been taught to accept an absolute distinction between body and soul, or matter and mind. For one thing, it is easier to make theories that way. Also, modern history has shown the astonishing success of material inventions; for most people in the West it does not appear that another philosophy is needed for progress. Additionally, for many, especially those with higher education, theology and similar thought that proposes that the soul is connected to god has lost its meaning. As a consequence, for these people discussion of mental substance has become meaningless. Today, most people tend to talk or write about only that which is measurable and which can be analyzed through science and instrumentation.

In reality, the scientific view that mind and body are separate does not agree with our daily experience. For instance, we often use inherently contradictory language when we ask "What's on your mind?" and are answered "It doesn't matter." Or likewise, we accept when "What's the matter," is answered by "Oh, never mind." We rarely reflect on how "scientifically" meaningless such daily exchanges are. They show how unified our thinking is, and how peculiar it is that in our scientific worldview we do not accept that fact of life. Actually, modern scientific experiments are beginning to show this shortcoming in our conventional body of knowledge, as we are (re)discovering the unity of life, and therefore the error of forcing mind apart from body. It has again become scientifically acceptable to study some of the indivisible relations between body and mind, perceived since the beginning of human history. Of course, Descartes knew of mind/body interactions, but his philosophy did not encourage their research. Only recently have the following fields of interaction been systematically explored:

Events Caused by Matter Influencing Mind Many substances influence the way our brains function. For instance, we know that deficiencies in minerals and vitamins and the pollution of food, water and air can cause mental disturbance (a hundred years ago in *A Christmas Carol* Charles Dickens wrote that Scrooge thought something in his evening meal made him see the ghosts of Christmas!). The mental illusions, hallucinations and delusions caused by LSD or angel dust are only too well known.

Experiences of Mind Influencing the Body Many psychological reasons for changes in physiological functions have been explored. One of the earliest challenges to the mind/body split proposed by Descartes was what we now call hypnosis, popularized by Anton Mesmer in the late eighteenth century. Today many instances of mind over matter are well established. Some deal with the ability of people to envision certain things happening to the body, such as stigmata, where one bleeds from those places in the body where Christ was wounded when crucified. Internationally known and widely photographed some fifty years ago, a German girl named Theresa Neumann would spontaneously bleed from hands, feet, and side each year at Easter. Hypnosis research has demonstrated the ability of people to produce blisters on their skin when told they were being touched by hot metal when in reality the object touching their skin was an ordinary pencil. In the most dramatic research to date, people with multiple personality disorders (MPD) have been shown to produce such personality-specific illness as asthma and even diabetes; these conditions appear and disappear depending upon which personality controls the MPD patient.

Knowledge of mental control over what happens to the body has led to what we know as psychosomatic medicine. It is now generally accepted that such diseases as gastric ulcer, asthma, and high blood pressure are greatly influenced by the state of mind. It even appears possible that certain physical diseases are the result of chronic stress. These results have led to an intensified search for specific psychological means to prevent the body's overreaction. The age-old technique of meditation has again come into fashion. And, as befits our modern fascination with gadgets, the technique of biofeedback has proved beneficial in the control of some illness. With the help of electronic signaling instrumentation, patients can learn to control their blood pressure and even more complex bodily functions. Likewise, visualization and guided mental imagery are proving effective in treating physical conditions.

Mixed Interactions It is not always clear if the body influences the mind, or the other way around, or if there is a mutual strengthening of body and mind. For instance, meditation combined with physical exercises has been shown to bring about relaxation, improved mental functioning, and athletic ability. It is in this area that the *connection* between mind/body techniques accepted in the West and Chinese chi gong can best be understood.

As we will discuss in chapter 13, recent developments in medicine in the West carry implicit acknowledgement of our vast ignorance in terms of how mind and matter interact. There is no doubt that the influence of mind on states of the body is firmly established, and Roger Sperry[5] has gone so far as to claim that the awareness of inner consciousness is "a causal reality." If we were to look at chi as the relationship which integrates the body (matter) and the mind (process), then the practice of chi gong, by heightening awareness, would understandably result in what the Chinese call "extraordinary human functions," or paranormal phenomena. But no matter how one looks at the mind/body connection, the study of chi phenomena cannot help but bring about a complete revision of conventional Western insights into the healing process.

How Do People of the West and of the East Think About Health?

The separation between modern Western and traditional Eastern thinking may well be illustrated by the differences in techniques of healing. We can use the following flowchart to clarify the difference.

In the	West	East
there is		
accent on	Body (matter)	Balance (mind-body)
	Disease as reaction	Disease as imbalanced energy
	Mechanistic analysis	Holistic analysis
	Material intervention	Creative rearrangement of
	(therapy)	*yin-yang*

People believe

energy enters through stomach and lungs to become:

	food for calories	food for *yin* or *yang*
	air for oxygen	breathing to activate chi
	pharmaceuticals, etc.	herbs with *yin-yang* qualities

and also enters through healing techniques:

	through circulation	through blood and chi
	(transfusion)	channels or yoga (Indian),
	or body cavities, or skin	chi gong, acupuncture, etc.

which are controlled by

	the nervous system	chakras (Indian) or acupoints
	transmitting messages by	and chi channels
	electricity or chemicals	accommodating the flow of
		vital energy

Disease is caused by

	malfunction of specific	lifestyle, our state of mind,
	organs or tissue, e.g.,	what we eat, do, etc.
	through environmental	
	influences	

The modern Western view of the functions of the body likens those to any process in a mechanistic universe: *Reaction* to outside forces is the most important aspect of life. The reactions of the body to the disease-causing agents in the environment can be grouped into typical patterns, which make for discrete diseases. And humans are perceived as essentially passive when it comes to "getting" a disease. Thus much of modern medicine is directed toward finding *external* causes for illness and little attention is given to what goes on in the patient's mind. This attitude of many Western doctors is reinforced because the general public often thinks that most of our actions are in response to environmental demands, and that the only thing our body needs to stay alive is fuel. Food is the fuel for the body motor. Air and additives (drugs, for instance) make the engine run better. When the body is sick, we go to a repair shop (hospital) and get it adjusted with more additives (medicines, extra blood or fluids, surgical implants, and so on). Yet, as Harvard professor Benson remarks: "at present only about 25 percent of the illnesses that bring a Western patient to a Western physician are successfully treated by specific agents and procedures."[6]

In the traditional Chinese view, *action*, evidenced by the fact that living organisms are characterized by movement, is foremost. The male (*yang*) and the female (*yin*) principles are kept in constant balance by one's own activity. This is not a mechanistic process, not just a reaction to what happens around us, but an active integration of body and mind functioning together. When one fails to maintain this balance one becomes ill. The actions of the body when ill reveal the places where the imbalance between *yin* and *yang* forces exist. The disturbances in balance may be due to many different types or aspects of chi, including "weakness" and "clogging," as described in the next chapter.

The ongoing process of maintaining health by balancing the *yin* and *yang* rests on the attention paid to circulating chi, the energy and information which balance the *yin* and *yang*. "Energy" and "information" are Western terms used to understand chi. Chi would include "calories," the source of physical energy (to sustain movement) in our materialistic philosophy. But it is much more. The difference can be illustrated with the example given by Professor Ralph G. H. Siu, contrasting the Western concept of physical energy and the life energy of chi:

> The unit of the calorie has been the primary measure of nutritional value. It has been used in great rigor in determining the energy relationships in an operating engine. A given process can be described in the number of calories absorbed or liberated. Calories can be employed in qualifying chemical reactions occurring in a living organism as it grows and in a dead organism as it decays. Exactly the same equations hold in both cases. Clearly then the term calorie does not describe the essence of living.[7]

It is obvious in Western science and medicine that movement in general (which common sense easily identifies as one difference between a living and a dead person) is not a prominent indicator of life and health, as it is in Chinese medicine.

The discussion of the importance of action (rather than reaction) in Chinese medicine brings us to another profound and mysterious aspect of chi. As we mention in chapter 1, chi also acts as a messenger and may foster exchange of information about the function of different organs and parts of the body. Chi is subtle or delicate as well, in that it can be concentrated or distributed by meditation and certain exercises (the practice of chi gong). In the West we have developed equivalents to some aspects of chi activation, for instance the use of massage to enhance or release energy. More to the point perhaps is the type of massage invented by Ida Rolfe; what is called structural integration or rolfing deals with muscle memories which bind energy. This comes close to the information content of chi.

How Do People of the West and of the East Manage Illness?

This brief description of the differences between modern medicine and the knowledge of methods to activate chi as an ancient way of healing is far from complete. But it may make it easier to understand which types of physical problems are more easily treated by each approach to health. Western medicine, because of the passive role of the patient, lends itself to treatment of acute illness, in which the patient may be unable to function at all or requires immediate assistance, especially in surgical cases. Chi gong (and the other branches of Chinese medicine as described in the next chapter), because it considers the active, or creative, role of patients, and views them as capable of restoring their own health, is more suited for the treatment of chronic conditions or disabilities, in which the patients have to find their own ways to live with illness.

One might think about the difference between the effectiveness of Eastern and Western medicine in terms of the mind/body interaction involved in different illnesses. Since Western science is based primarily on the study of the material body, it is best suited for those occasions when the body is suddenly incapacitated, when mental functioning has had little time to adapt to the disability. For instance, when consciousness is lost in an accident, one would not be able to participate in the healing technique. In acute illness the mind/body interaction is therefore not always of primary importance, and knowledge in this area is less necessary for the healer. However, if the condition is chronic, one clearly is capable of "minding it." We all know examples of adaptation to sickness by changing diet, lifestyle, or attitude. Since Chinese traditional science does not differentiate between mind and matter, it is to be expected that it would be better suited to dealing with any necessary adaptation to chronic illness.

This distinction in healing techniques does not mean that the

West has not developed cures for chronic illness or that Chinese traditional medicine is powerless in acute illness. In China today both types of medicine are practiced, and we look forward to the day when Western society incorporates a similar balance of Eastern and Western healing.

In China, all centers of population have modern hospitals with emergency rooms and medical-surgical facilities. In addition there are many practitioners of traditional medicine with specialists in herbal treatment and other Chinese pharmacological methods, as well as specialists in all varieties of acupuncture. Moreover, when Dr. Esser discussed medical training at the Beijing College of Traditional Chinese Medicine, he was told that *all* Chinese doctors are trained in both Western and traditional Chinese concepts. The Western medical schools devote approximately four days per week to the study of modern medicine and one day to traditional medicine. In the schools of traditional Chinese medicine it is the other way around. As we have described, the chi gong training for health, as well as the direct treatment for certain diseases by a chi gong master, is another method available for healing in China. In chapter 4 we will share our observations of how this Chinese modern-traditional health system works and review some of its results.

In Guangzhou, Paul Dong talked with some patients who were seeking external chi treatment from a chi gong master. "Without a doctor's diagnosis, how can one determine what the ailment is?" asked Dong. "A doctor's diagnosis is not always correct," replied a female patient. "The important thing is that one knows what one's own illness is" (and therefore can determine whether chi would help). A male patient added that even a minor ailment could turn into a major one if one had to wait for hours to get help. The chi gong master who was applying external chi then joined in: "We know the principles of *jinglou* [the network of channels through which the chi energy circulates] and that's why there can be no serious problem. Of course, minor errors are inevitable." After a pause he continued: "We only accept ordinary cases for treatment. If it is a serious case, we usually suggest that the patient be examined at a hospital before we accept him or her for treatment. And," he added, "of course there is nothing we can do if the patient refuses to have a medical examination."

Types of Chi Healing

There are three ways to use chi gong for therapeutic purposes. First, there is the external chi therapy. Second is self-training— choosing a chi gong course and performing the exercises properly can prove effective within one hundred days. Third, there is the combination of the two: receiving external chi treatment in addition to doing chi gong exercises and thereby strengthening the therapeutic effect of both.

There are three ways of applying external chi therapy. The first involves sending chi directly at the focus of the affliction, just as Dong did when treating his wife's chest lump. The second way releases chi along *jinglou,* the network of bodily energy channels. Third is applying the treatment at a selected acupoint for the disorder. Whichever method is chosen, it is based on the same principles as acupuncture. External chi practitioners know in general the network of channels and the acupoints for various diseases. But some novices, ignorant of the position of the channels, can also achieve results by using focal treatment alone. (Because an error may be dangerous, we advise against such experimentation.) For once chi enters the body, it will automatically travel along the route of the channels to reach every part of the body, including the focus of affliction. This is also the reason that when one ailment is being treated, other ailments often are cured at the same time. This phenomenon occurs with acupuncture as well.

External chi treatment is not helpful for everyone. In Dong's experience one in four persons experiences excellent results, while half of the patients show significant improvement, and the remainder some or none at all. There seem to be degrees to which persons are susceptible to external chi; probably their responsiveness is related to inherited traits (in the way some people are susceptible to becoming intoxicated with a small amount of wine and others have a very high tolerance for alcohol).

However, there are ways to strengthen the response. For instance, when acupuncture is ineffective, the addition of external chi may make the difference. After the needles are inserted, a doctor who also practices external chi can increase the curative effect. Dr. Chen Yin-long, the superintendent of the School of Traditional Chinese Medicine in Xiamen (Amoy), is known as a miracle doctor because he uses this technique in treating his patients. Chen is a chi gong master of the *linzi* technique, having practiced for thirty years. *Linzi*, which literally means "moving spirit," is a Japanese chi gong technique.

When a chi gong master releases his or her energy, the patient may show signs of being activated, as in the chi gong term, "activated by external chi." Take for example the treatment Dong gave his wife for her cold symptom of a stuffed nose. He directed his external chi to her nose and in the process her head sometimes shook uncontrollably and incessantly. The famous chi gong master Huang Rui-sin at the Jujian Provincial Hospital of Traditional Chinese Medicine in Hangchow is known for his activation by external chi. He usually issues his chi at a distance of over one foot from the patient. In demonstrations he would often release his chi from about ten feet away and still cause the patient to shake vigorously.[8]

A doctor of Traditional Chinese Medicine has to be a chi gong practitioner to be able to apply external chi. However, not every chi gong practitioner can generate external chi. This appears to depend on the type of chi gong one practices. For health care and self-treatment it usually takes about one hundred days for chi gong exercises to show their effect. It may take a year to experience improvement in one's own disease. But achieving release of external chi requires years of training and depends on what type of skill one is aiming for. For certain types of external chi even ten years of training may not be enough (see chapters 8 and 9). Generally speaking, it is easier to acquire external chi by training in the Movement Skill Exercise of chi gong. Paul Dong, ignorant at first of the best training procedures, practiced the Static Skill Exercise (relaxed and quiet chi gong) for four years without succeeding in the release of external chi. Later he switched to the Movement Skill and began feeling the chi. He then supplemented this training with Standing-On-Stake (which will be discussed in chapter 8).

Many people, including students in Dong's chi gong class at the San Francisco China Town YMCA, have asked if external chi therapy is the same as psychic healing. Dong does not think so. Although some psychic healers describe their work in terms of energy transfer, the transfer of chi may be a different aspect of the mind/body complex. There also may be different types of psychic healers. Christian Science practitioners and New Thought remote healers often work at a distance, sometimes many miles. This may overlap with some types of chi energy, which can and do transfer over distance (see the discussion of infrasonics in chapter 1 and of Empty Force in chapter 6), but presumably, what operates in psychic healing is one's thought, whereas external chi is bioenergy, which in some manifestations can be measured. The life energy is possessed by everyone, but only becomes vigorous when activated by a chi gong master or through intensive personal chi gong training. This energy is stored in the body and can be released by certain methods. In skill training one clears the network of internal channels and chooses a sensitive part of the body (the *laogong* acupoint or fingertips) to release the chi (see chapter 9). It appears that this process is 90 percent energy and 10 percent thought; chi gong masters typically feel somewhat exhausted after providing external chi treatment because they have expended some of their energy. Therefore chi gong masters usually limit the number of patients they see each day to four or five.

Dr. Wang Ying, in his *External Qi Therapy of Qi Gong*[9], points to the following characteristics of healing by a chi gong master:

1. Therapeutic effects have often been obtained in cases where other treatments by Western or Chinese traditional medicine principles have had poor results. Additionally, relapses occur less often in cases cured by external chi treatment.

2. Patients cured by external chi treatment feel "easy" and "comfortable" in the treated area or area of affliction. After several consecutive treatments patients improve in terms of spirit, appetite, sleep, and complexion.

3. The response to external chi treatment depends not so much on the nature of the disease as on the degree of the patient's receptivity to chi. If the patient has good receptivity, external chi can be effective even in complicated cases. One might say that patients with a sensitive network of internal chi channels show good results with external chi treatment.

4. Diseases can be cured and at the same time the constitution of the patient can be improved by external chi treatment.

5. External chi treatment can cure several disordered conditions in the patient all at the same time.

6. Clinical practice indicates that external chi treatment can relieve pain, allay inflammation, diminish tumors, kill cancer cells, and enhance the immune function of the body. It also resists rheumatism, stops muscular atrophy, and promotes general metabolism.

7. External chi treatment is simple and convenient. It can be performed in any place and does not require equipment or

medication. It may be applied to young and old, man or woman.

We cannot be certain at this point that all such claims can be verified. However, Dr. Wang's list shows the importance of the concept of chi in the prevention and healing of a large part of human suffering. We want to show that as effective as external chi treatment is purported to be, it cannot be considered other than as a temporary measure in treatment. The basic way for maintaining health and treating certain disorders is one's own practice of chi gong.

Notes

1. Ren Ying-qin as quoted in: David Eisenberg, *Encounters with Qi: Exploring Chinese Medicine* (New York: Penguin, 1987), 90.

2. Paul Dong only applies external chi after the person in need has been examined by a licensed M.D. and referral for chi gong has been made.

3. See: Bruce Holbrook, *The Stone Monkey: An Alternative Chinese-Scientific Reality* (New York: William Morrow, 1981).

4. As Larry Dossey, M.D., pointed out, one might argue that Descartes also tried for unity by postulating the pineal gland in the brain as the region for transactions between the body and mind (which has recently become plausible with the discovery of neuropeptides, many of which are from the pineal, see chap. 13). But Dr. Dossey also emphasizes that "dualism of mind and body is a dominant force in modern medical theory." Larry Dossey, *Beyond Illness: Discovering the Experience of Health* (Boston: Shambala, 1985), 14.

5. Roger Sperry, one of the foremost researchers of the split brain, has formulated a "new mental paradigm," which postulates that mental, not physical, forces constitute the top of the hierarchy of brain control. See Roger Sperry in *Perspectives in Biology and Medicine* 29 (1987): 413–22. Similarly, Nobel laureate and neurophysiologist Sir John Eccles, building on the observations of Wilder Penfield, the great Canadian neurosurgeon, and Roger Sperry, has stated that mind is primary and acts on the brain.

6. Eisenberg, *Encounters with Qi*, 13. Even worse, F. J. Ingelfinger, M.D., the late editor of the authoritative *New England Journal of Medicine*, has said that in only 10 percent of patients can modern medical intervention be considered dramatically successful, while perhaps 80 percent of patients have either self-limiting disorders or conditions that cannot be improved—in *New England Journal of Medicine* 296 (1977): 448–49. Dr.

Ingelfinger later expressed this in other terms, in his posthumously printed George W. Gay lecture, delivered at Harvard Medical School. There he quoted the general figure "90 percent of the visits by patients to doctors are caused by conditions that are either self-limited or beyond the capabilities of medicine"—see: *New England Journal of Medicine* 303 (1980): 1509.

7. Ralph G. H. Siu, *Chi: A Neo-Taoist Approach to Life* (Cambridge, Mass.: M.I.T. Press, 1974), 260.

8. This is the same as the spontaneous movement caused by bursts of circulating chi during the practice of advanced chi gong, as described in chapter 8.

9. Wang Ying, *External Qi Therapy of Qi Gong* (Tai Jeng: Shansi Provincial Publishing House for Science and Education, 1987).

3

The Role of Chi in Chi Gong, Acupuncture, and Herbal Medicine

The occurrence of disease is due to insufficiently balanced chi.
—*The Yellow Emperor's Classic of Internal Medicine*

The concept of chi as vital energy plays a role in all aspects of Chinese life. Thus it is to be expected that chi gong, as a natural way to maintain health and improve capabilities of body and mind, is practiced by many. At a 1984 chi gong conference in Xi'an, The People's Republic of China, which Paul Dong attended, professionals from all aspects of Chinese medicine, public health, sports, and the martial arts were among those taking part. One of the topics of discussion was "Who rules chi gong?"

For quite a few years there has been controversy throughout China over chi gong's rightful governance. After chi gong became popular, the Chinese medical community insisted that chi gong belonged to the province of traditional Chinese medicine (TCM), sports professionals stated that chi gong came under the heading of sports, and the fields of martial arts (because gong fu—special ability—is focal to them) and public health (because it deals with prevention) claimed chi gong for their disciplines.

Yang Xiao-wu, general secretary of the Guangdong Province Chi

Gong Scientific Research Association told Paul Dong, during a visit to Guanzhou, that he knew first hand of the controversy over who would govern chi gong. However, he treated the subject with humor, saying, "We will have the utmost respect for the leader of chi gong and go on doing our own things." (What he meant was, whoever wins the right to claim chi gong can have the honor, but cannot have any real power over those practitioners who develop chi gong further.)

Since ancient times the theory of chi as a basic vital force has been a part of TCM. Only since chi gong's recent rise in popularity have different fields decided to claim part of the heritage and share the glory. That sports and martial arts claim chi gong as their own results from a convoluted argument. It is like placing the cart before the horse, because without first practicing chi gong, martial arts practitioners and athletes would not have the inner strength necessary for their disciplines. Likewise, the claim of public health professionals to be responsible for the development of chi gong is exaggerated. Public health is concerned primarily with external cleanliness and preventive measures, which have little to do with training the inner body/mind of the individual.

While the different disciplines are in dispute over primacy, the fact is chi gong's origin stems from ancient Chinese medicine, perhaps as much as five thousand years ago. The practice of chi gong was first systematically described approximately two thousand years ago in *The Yellow Emperor's Classic of Internal Medicine*. [1] Today, medicine is very much the driving force in the development of scientific knowledge of chi. For instance, the preliminary agreement for cooperative research on chi gong between the U.S. and China concluded in 1987 took place via medical schools (Cambridge Hospital, affiliated with Harvard Medical School, and the Beijing College of Traditional Chinese Medicine, see chapter 11). The First World Conference for Academic Exchange of Medical Chi Gong in Beijing,

October 10–13, 1988, also came under the aegis of medicine. The six countries with official representation at this conference, China, the U.S., Italy, France, Japan, and Australia expressed the unanimous opinion that chi gong is a medical discipline.

What Did the Ancient Chinese Believe About the Relationships Between Chi and Health?

Chinese medicine pays great attention to prevention. Historically, in the practice of traditional Chinese medicine physicians would only be paid when the patient remained healthy. If he or she became ill, payment would stop until recovery occurred. A famous line from *The Emperor's Classic* states: "Sophisticated medicine treats future diseases; crude medicine cures present diseases." Chinese physicians today maintain that preventing disease is more important than curing diseases, and one should not wait for illness to strike before one practices medicine. The most important goal in practicing chi gong is the prevention of disease (maintenance of health) and the support of the life organism.[2] It is therefore understandable that the ancient Chinese devoted much thought to the different forms of chi in nature and how humans can benefit from this knowledge.

The concept of chi (energy, air, information) is found throughout many ancient Chinese medical texts. Of course, chi in Chinese medicine includes the air found in nature, but it refers more often to chi inside the body. For example, *The Emperor's Classic* states, "*True chi* comes from the heavens, and is further nourished by *acquired chi* which fills the body." That is to say, a person's true chi, the vital force of life, is composed of *yuan* chi (original chi), which exists when a person is born, and *jing* chi (circulating along the meridians, see chapter 1). Simply put, a person's vital force must be propelled by true chi, and the strength or weakness of the true chi will affect the strength or weakness of the vital force. Furthermore, the term *original chi* also includes two aspects, original *yin* and original *yang*, which come from one's parents. These are focused in the *ming men* (gate of vitality—an area in the back, between the kidneys), and the *dan tian* (an area in the front, below the navel) respectively. Original chi is the wellspring of vital action. We are born with original chi; how do we *acquire* chi later?

Acquired chi comes from such substances as food and water. After this material undergoes biochemical processes inside the body, it forms "material vital quintessence," also known as nourishment chi, or *jing* chi. *The Emperor's Classic* says, "Nourishment chi in the body includes secretions and body fluids, and when it enters the arteries, it becomes part of the bloodstream and brings nourishment to the ends of the limbs and the internal organs."

Another source of acquired chi is the air. Modern medical science divides the breathing processes of the body into two parts, external breathing (breathing through the lungs) and internal breathing (cell respiration). The entire process is as follows:

The lungs admit air (exchanging carbon dioxide for the oxygen in natural air).
→ Hemoglobin in the red blood corpuscles combines with the oxygen.
→ The oxygen is transported to all organs via the circulation of the blood.
→ Cell structure oxidation and metabolism produce carbon dioxide which is passed back to the blood.
→ Carbon dioxide passes from the bloodstream into the lungs to be exhaled from the body.

For Westerners this fully describes the process by which man and nature exchange gases. In Chinese medicine, which very strongly emphasizes the relationship between man and nature, the exchange of chi is considered in addition to that of oxygen. Long ago, *The Emperor's Classic* brought up the theory of "the unity of man and nature." Chinese medicine considers humans to be one of the myriad works of nature, which cannot be separated from the natural environment. Obviously the relationship between humans and air is vital; to stop breathing is to end one's life. Therefore, Chinese medicine considers the practice of chi gong to be a most basic step in the promotion of health.

Chinese medicine considers the greatest influence on the body to be the natural variations of the weather. The four seasons in a year found in nature, with seasonal changes going through hot, cold, warm, and cool phases, are called *si shi* (the four periods) in Chinese medicine. In addition, during the four seasons of the year, the atmosphere goes through the six conditions of wind, cold, heat, dampness, dryness, and fire, caused by the changing seasons. In normal cases, these changes are called *liu chi* (the six atmospheres), and in abnormal cases they are called *liu yin* (the six evils). The six evils are caused by sudden and abnormally large variations in temperature, humidity, or other atmospheric factors. When these bring about imbalance of *yin* and *yang* in the body, disease results.

The body's ability to cope with the elements also undergoes changes in accordance with the changes in the four periods and the six atmospheres. The likelihood that the six evils will cause disease is related to the strength or weakness of the true chi. When the true chi is strong, the body can resist the assaults of the six evils.

Acquired chi of the yin type is from the Earth and is concentrated in the *ming men* area. The yang type of acquired chi is primarily collected in the *bai hui* acupoint on the crown of the head. Coming from the heavens, this chi goes to the *dan tian* area. *The Emperor's Classic* says, "Solar [yang] chi from the heavens flows down to the earth, and [water] vapor from the earth ascends. The vapor[3] stirs in the heavens, and thus what is high is met from below, and what is rising [water vapor] is interchanged with what is falling [rain]!" And further: "Movement and stillness meet, above and below intersect, yin and yang intermingle, and life is made from their changes." This means that the universe is not static; it is in constant motion. Because the solar chi from the heavens falls, the water vapor from the earth rises. This continuous state of flux gives rise to all change, and this change produces the infinite variety of things we observe on earth. Humans live in the midst of this constant exchange of air between the heavens and the earth, and are the product of such changes. *The Emperor's Classic* further states, "Man is born on the earth and dies in the heavens. Heaven and earth share the same ch'i, and man has life.[4] One who can withstand the four periods, who has heaven and earth for parents, and who knows the myriad of things, is called the son of heaven."

Chinese medicine revealed the following pattern in the four periods and the six atmospheres: "spring rules birth, summer rules growth, autumn rules gathering, and winter rules storing" (*The Emperor's Classic*). The method of maintaining health should vary with the changing of the four periods and the six atmospheres. The principle to remember is that according to ancient wisdom healthy activities should be consonant with the functions of the seasons: spring sustains birth, summer sustains growth, autumn sustains gathering, and winter sustains storing. And what is more, Chinese medicine even divides human activities of day and night into four parts, i.e., dawn sustains birth, midday sustains growth, dusk sustains gathering, and night sustains storing. We can compare the application of different principles governing parts of a day or the year to what is known in Western science as diurnal and seasonal rhythms.

Chinese medicine refers to the body's ability to resist disease (we might call it the immune system) as *wei* chi (protective or defensive chi), because it protects the body and resists the attacks of external ills. The level of strength of protective chi is also intimately related to the adequacy of the supply of nourishment chi. When nourishment chi is sufficient, protective chi flourishes.

The opposite of protective chi is *ill* chi. Ill chi refers mainly to the six evils, and it is a disease-causing agent. *The Emperor's Classic* formulates this as, "When the good chi [true chi] lies within, the evil can do nothing." And further, "Wind, rain, cold, and heat are not insubstantial, and one who suddenly encounters a burst of wind and heavy rain but doesn't get sick is not empty, and so those ills cannot harm that person."

Evidently, in order to promote longevity it is necessary to strengthen the body's ability to withstand the natural environment. Chi gong is an important method of enhancing this endurance. The practice of chi gong is not the same as modern body-building exercises. Chinese medicine brings up the question of the relationship of "form" to "spirit." Form refers to physical form, that is, the body, the physique. Spirit refers to the spiritual, psychological, and mental side of the person. Modern body-building exercises concentrate on the exercise of the muscles and overlook the importance of spirit. In contrast, the ancient practice of chi gong emphasizes the need for a sound mind in a sound body, that is, the need for body-building exercises to pay serious attention to activating the spirit and activating the mind. Similarly, for the ancient Romans, *Mens sana in corpora sano* (a sound mind in a sound body) was of the essence. *The Emperor's Classic* promises, "With a sound mind in a sound body, a person can live out a full life-span and go on living for a hundred years until dying." Further, "Form is the house of spirit, and spirit is lord to form." That is to say, the body [form] provides the spirit with a base [house] in which to exist, while the spirit lords over the body in the sense that the physical form follows the orders of the spirit. For this reason, the practice of chi gong not only exercises the body, but also exercises the spirit—the psychological, spiritual and mental state.

Chi in Acupuncture, Herbal Medicine, and Chi Gong

All aspects of traditional Chinese medicine are based on the concept of the circulation of chi. This is as important as the circulation of blood, and problems in balancing different types of chi and their circulation cause disease. Ways of ensuring that the chi remains balanced and circulates well are countless, but the main specialties for the treatment of diseases in TCM are the different forms of acupuncture, herbology or herbal medicine, chi gong, massage, and dietetics (the prevention of disease by proper nutrition). We will not discuss the latter two specialties since they are beyond the scope of this book and add relatively little to understanding the ancient theories of chi.

Chinese herbology, acupuncture, and chi gong are three parts of a single entity, as closely related as water, steam, and ice. They can be and often are used separately, and may be used together. With dietetics and massage they are considered to be the indispensable components of traditional Chinese health care. Almost three thousand years ago, *The Emperor's Classic* explained their applications and functions in detail. While acupuncture and herbal medicine typically focus on curing sickness, chi gong usually focuses on maintaining good health (as do massage and balanced—for *yin* and *yang*—nutrition).

The preceding brief description of some aspects of the concept of chi in Chinese medicine may give us insight into the rationale for different chi-based treatments. Herbal medicine and acupuncture are most often used by the patient who actively suffers from symptoms of a disease, because they fulfill the role of "temporary cures" by restoring the *yin/yang* balance. As we emphasize throughout this book, the best way to health is maintaining the balance of *yin* and *yang* through a proper life-style, dietary measures, and chi gong. However, if one is seriously ill, often the practice of chi gong is impossible and thus one can only begin to maintain good health after the balance of *yin/yang* is restored (temporarily) with acupuncture, herbs, or massage.

Turning first to a discussion of acupuncture: Its meridian (channel) system is an invisible network that allows *yin* and *yang* chi to enter into the body fluid circulation. Each meridian is said to correspond to a specific internal organ (e.g., heart, lung, kidney) where energy is stored or generated depending on the time of day and the season. The primary purpose of acupuncture is to correct any energy disturbance or blockage in the meridian network that may cause disease. Acupuncture restores the energy balance by moving the chi, that is, stimulating it in places if there is deficiency, or releasing it if there is excess. The practice of chi gong is the *active control* of the chi's movement in the body, while acupuncture is a way to *passively* promote the movement of the chi and blood in the body. Scientific evidence of this "movement" has been provided by infrared detectors on the skin, which show increased temperature in areas affected by acupuncture.[5] Chinese medicine asserts that many diseases are caused by obstruction of the smooth flow of chi and blood. It is thought that all aches are due to a clogging of chi and blood, and so it is said that "If it's held stuck it hurts, and if it flows freely it's fine." Therefore, acupuncture emphasizes gaining chi in curing disease and requires chi reaching the locus of disease. If the patient has no sense of gaining chi, the effectiveness of the cure will be reduced, even so far as to have no effectiveness. "Gaining chi" is evidenced by sole or combined feelings of sourness, swelling, heaviness, and numbness. Manipulating the needle by hand, it is possible to transmit what is felt at the point of the needle insertion through the lines of the meridians to the locus of disease.[6] For example, needling the *zu san li*, an acupuncture point on the lower leg, can cure gastralgia (stomach pains). When the needle pierces the *zu san li*, at first there is a local feeling of gaining chi, and after performing a twisting motion with the needle, the chi flows up to the stomach. This is what is meant by "chi reaching the locus of disease."

Recognition of the efficacy of acupuncture was provided in a 1979 report of the World Health Organization, which concluded that "acupuncture must be taken seriously as a clinical procedure of considerable value." At that time, a list of forty diseases that could be effectively treated by acupuncture was compiled. [7]

According to the annals, many ancient Chinese doctors practiced chi gong. For this reason, ancient Chinese medical texts on acupuncture provide a large number of examples of the combined use of chi gong and acupuncture, with such names as Needle Method Without Steps and Needle Method of the Unity of Mind and Chi. All these acupuncture techniques refer to an acupuncture master (who is also a chi gong master). The master makes use of the hands as well as the needle to transmit his own internal chi into the meridians and acupuncture points of the patient. In this way, he regulates the patient's *jing* chi (meridian chi) and achieves the goal of curing the disease. This technique requires an outstanding virtuoso of acupuncture, of a kind rarely seen in modern clinical practice. Performing this procedure demands a great deal of energy from the chi gong master.

Activating Chi in the Small and Large Circuits Every Chinese practitioner of chi gong has heard of the *small circuit* and the *large circuit*. This is a shared feature of chi gong and medical theory. The small circuit (also called *microcosmic cycle* or *orbit*) and the large circuit (also called *heavenly cycle*) circulate the chi respectively through the central (front and rear) meridians of our body trunk, and through all the twelve meridians, including circulation through the extremities.

The student will master the circulation through the small circuit first, in about one year of chi gong practice. The small circuit consists of the functional channel (or meridian) running in front of the body from the top of the head to the perineum, and the governing channel, running at the back of the body from the perineum to the crown of the head.

The governing channel is particularly important for *yang* energy (male, light, from the heavens) while the functional channel is the main conduit for the *yin* energy (female, dark, from the earth). When the small circuit is engaged there is a feeling of warmth moving down from below the navel (*dan tian*) to the perineum (*hui-yin* or "port of mortality," halfway between the external sex organs and the anus), then up along the spine through the area between the kidneys, opposite the navel (*ming men* or "gate of vitality," collector of *yin* energy) to the crown of the head (*bai-hui*, collector of *yang* energy). From there the chi will move down via the breastbone (*san-chung*, "heart" point, midway between the nipples) back to the navel. The circuit will be activated automatically once the student practices chi gong regularly. There has been no explanation in ancient or modern times why the circulation of the chi goes in this particular manner and not the other way around. But the engagement of the small circuit testifies to the fact that the blood and chi are flowing smoothly throughout the body (see fig. 3-1).

Two or three years after mastering the small circuit, the student will experience activation of the large circuit, provided that he or she continues to practice a sufficient amount of time each day (see chapters 8 and 9). The large circuit spreads the feeling of warmth all over the body, including the hands and the feet (see fig. 3-2), as well as the internal organs. Important acupoints on the routes of these additional channels or meridians are the *yong quan* point (part of the kidney meridian, located on the sole of the foot) and the *laogong* point (part of the pericardium meridian, located in the middle of the palm). Once the chi gong practitioner experiences engagement of the large circuit, he or she is assured of a very strong flow of chi and blood, and therefore good health and longevity.

This process of circulation of chi in the small and large circuits is

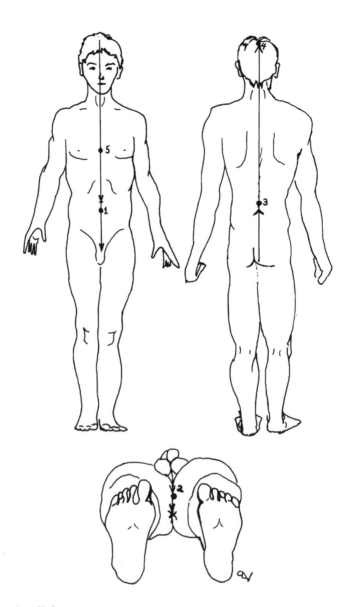

The Small Circuit

When the small circuit is activated, chi flows from acupoints 1 through 5 and then returns to 1, the *dan tian*. Please realize that the lines representing the governing (in the back) and the functional (in the front) meridians are not located on the surface of the body—the acupoints are also not located on the skin itself.

70

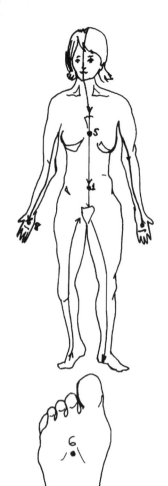

Key for Figures 3-1 and 3-2

Acupoints	1	Dan Tian
	2	Hui-Yin
	3	Ming Men
	4	Bai-hui
	5	San-Chung
	6	Yong Quan
	7	Dazhui
	8	Laogong

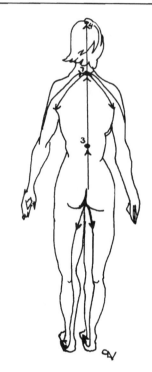

The Large Circuit

When the large circuit is activated, chi flows from the *dan tian* to *hui-yin* (point 2 on the perineum). It then travels first to the feet, to return through point 6 (*yong quan* on the sole of the foot), to *hui-yin* and only then up the governing meridian to the *dazhui* point (7, in the nape of the neck). From there it will circulate through the arms via the *laogong* point (8, in the palm of the hand) back to *dazhui*. Only then will it complete the circuit, as in the case of the small circuit, via the *bai-hui* point along the functional meridian back to the *dan tian*.

71

at the root of the therapeutic principles by which acupuncture cures disease. Piercing the acupuncture points with needles will smooth the disturbed or obstructed flow of chi and blood and stimulates movement through the meridians or channels.

Herbal Medicine As for the relationship between Chinese herbal medicine and chi gong, we can offer only a brief discussion here. Superficially it may appear that herbal medicine is similar to Western pharmaceutics, the only difference being that the Chinese deal with traditional concepts of the healing properties of plants, and to a lesser degree animal and mineral substances. Although the classical and medieval Western "herbals," or descriptions of the medicinal properties of plants, are similar, perhaps nowhere is the difference between modern Western and Chinese approaches to medicine greater than in the medical use of materials entering our body.

The study of Chinese herbal medicine begins with an understanding of the *yin* and *yang* properties of food and the medicinal properties of herbs. For instance, the properties of all herbs in Chinese medicine are classified according to the four atmospheres and the five flavors. The four atmospheres are the cold, hot, warm, and cool characteristics of herbal medicine, also called the four properties. The five flavors refer to both taste and odor, according to the human senses. They are classified as spicy, sweet, sour, bitter, and salty. The four atmospheres (or properties) and the five flavors are considered in combination. For example, cold herbs may be further classified as bitter cold and sweet cold, and sweet herbs as warm sweet and cold sweet.

A certain formula or combination of herbs can have diverse effects, such as fortifying the lungs, the spleen, the kidney, the chi, and the blood. After entering the body, the medicine passes through the channels and meridians to the internal organs. Each herb is known chiefly to enter and affect one or more of certain meridians and subsequently the organs and functions associated with them. Here we see again that Chinese herbal medicine, chi gong, and acupuncture are alike, in that all achieve their healing effects by promoting the passage of chi through the meridians to the internal organs.

The primary therapeutic effects of Chinese herbal medicine are to change the flows and qualities of chi, and since chi governs blood, affect blood circulation. The effects of Chinese herbal medicine on chi can be divided into the two categories of *fortifying the chi* and *stirring up the chi*. Chinese medicine teaches that the main pathologies of chi are feeble chi and clogged chi. The principle for treating these pathologies is: Fortifying the chi is good for feeble chi, and stirring up the chi is good for clogged chi.

It is not hard to understand that chi may be feeble, as we ourselves know that our energies can run low due to many diverse causes. One might think of fortifying the chi as similar to taking food or medication to strengthen oneself, and indeed in cases of feeble chi dietetics may be used in addition to herbal remedies to treat diseases.

The symptoms of clogged chi (rather than excess chi) are probably most commonly seen in clinical practice. For example, problems of the stomach, swelling of the abdominal cavity, constipation of the bowels and difficulties urinating, or an irregular menstrual cycle all may be caused by clogged chi. There are a large number of Chinese herbal remedies for stirring up the chi.

It can be said that for all Chinese herbal medicine the principles of fortifying the chi, stirring up the chi, regulating the chi, and so on, are the same as those used in chi gong to cure disease.

All facets of Chinese medicine complement each other and form a working unit. Acupuncture and herbal medicine tend more toward curing sickness, and chi gong tends more toward maintaining good health. In clinical practice, appropriate combinations of acupuncture plus herbs; acupuncture plus chi gong; herbs plus chi gong; or acupuncture plus chi gong plus herbs are applied depending on the physical condition of the patient.

Notes

1. I. Veith, trans., *The Yellow Emperor's Classic of Internal Medicine*, 2d ed. (Berkeley: Univ. of California Press, 1972).

2. *The Emperor's Classic* also says: "The sages did not treat those who were already ill; they instructed those who were not yet ill."

3. Solar chi is used in the sense of vapor which contains heat from the sun. *

4. Heavenly/solar chi (*yang*) corresponds to the heart and fire/heat; earthly chi (*yin*) corresponds to the kidneys and water. These are the two basic fetal organs, described as "heaven and earth in humans."

5. For instance, as proven in experiments by Mathew Lee, M.D., and Monique Ernst, M.D., Ph.D., described in "Clinical and Research Observations on Acupuncture Analgesia and Thermography," in *Scientific Bases of Acupuncture*, ed. Bruce Pomeranz and Gabriel Stux (New York: Springer-Verlag, 1989).

6. To express this more precisely, it is not the feeling that is spread, but it is feeling the movement of true chi going toward or coming from the locus.

7. R. H. Bannerman, *World Health Organization Viewpoint on Acupuncture*, published in 1979 and reprinted in *The American Journal of Acupuncture* 8 (1980): 231.

4

The Chi Gong Clinic

Primum nil nocere (*First, do no harm*)

Within three years of chi gong becoming popular in China, numerous chi gong hospitals and clinics sprang up, with more and more opening each year. [1] The number of chi gong facilities in the whole of China has probably reached more than a hundred by now. The explosive rise of the chi gong clinic is mainly due to China's huge population of one billion and the shortage of doctors and medicine.

It is not easy to understand how different ways of treatment in China exist beside one another, or how the Chinese decide whether a disorder should be treated with Western scientific medicine, with traditional Chinese medicine (TCM) or perhaps with a combination of both. Then, within TCM there are different approaches, which are traditionally used for different types of illness. Using present-day comparative research methods, all the approaches used in TCM treatments have been proven effective.

In the past decades, the widespread use of acupuncture has been encouraged by the Chinese government. Herbal medicine and massage are also available in the major traditional Chinese medicine hospitals. This eases to some extent the need for Western medical care, but the interminably long lines snaking out in front of hospital outpatient clinics still mean long waiting periods for all but the richest patients seeking diagnosis and treatment. Figures show approximately 557,000 available doctors trained in Western medicine in 1982 and 303,000 in TCM (Eisenberg, 1987). This is about 1 physician for 1,100 people, as compared to about 1 for 500 people in the U.S. For this reason the demand for chi gong is urgent. Its application consists of two methods of medical assistance: (1) learning a chi gong exercise, which takes only three to five days before patients can practice chi gong themselves to improve health or prevent disease; and (2) a chi gong expert applying external chi to try to cure the patient's disease. Chi gong experts can produce external chi after a minimum of one year of practicing chi gong, if they exercise intensely for many hours daily. This is one to two years less than the training period for an acupuncturist, three to five years less than that for a specialist in traditional Chinese medicine and many years less than the training period for a Western-style doctor.

At present, the largest chi gong hospital has three hundred hospital beds, and the smallest may have only ten beds. Chi gong clinics normally admit only fairly serious cases and will provide outpatient services for patients with common ailments. Because of the vast number of patients with the latter, an increasing number of chi gong specialists are opening private practices, with external chi treatment as their main service.

According to preliminary surveys, chi gong treatment has absorbed 15 percent of the patient load; traditional Chinese medicine, 15 percent; acupuncture, 27 percent; and the remaining 43 percent are taken care of by Western scientific medicine. There is a similarity between these figures and those of patients seeking relief in Western countries. For instance, in the U.S., approximately half of the patients of a general practitioner suffer from ailments without an identifiable organic base, that is, the available Western techniques do not lead to a meaningful diagnosis in such patients; 50 percent seems to be about the percentage of Chinese patients not served by Western scientific medicine.

Every country, no matter where, relies on Western scientific medicine as the main treatment for physically identifiable diseases, and China is no exception. We know that Western medicine is especially successful in the diagnosis and treatment of acute disorders, such as trauma, surgical emergencies, nonviral infectious diseases, and early diagnosable medical illness. In chronic conditions, and in those diseases where the patient complains of symptoms without demonstrable changes in organs or tissues, TCM appears to have good results. In this manner TCM can be said to complement Western medicine, and TCM is apparently also effective in many of the diseases caused by viruses, such as the common cold or flu. The experience of Paul Dong related at the beginning of chapter 2 also points in this direction.

In the past twenty years, China has tried to put forward a combination of Chinese and Western medicine. In certain facilities a systematic attempt has been made to use Western medicine for conditions that Chinese medicine cannot treat, and to turn to TCM for conditions where use of Western medicine is not satisfactory. Among the latter, the Chinese point to such chronic conditions as osteoarthritis, asthma, emphysema, ulcerative colitis, diabetes, etc. Alternatively, Chinese and Western medicine can be applied at the same time. If the results are not good enough, then acupuncture may be combined with them to provide a comprehensive treatment. Because of its present popularity, chi gong is also used as part of the combination. The results of using multiple treatment approaches are difficult to evaluate as there remains a rivalry and mistrust of each other's treatment methods in most of the doctors, whether practicing TCM or Western medicine. However, increasing exchange of data is expected to improve this situation (see chapter 11).

There is another reason to opt for a wide-ranging approach to medical problems. We know that many of the Western techniques of intervention carry risks, as shown by the mortality rates of operations and undesirable side effects of drugs. In the past decades, the increasing popularity in the West of (bio)behavioral medicine or stress reduction methods indicates the public's growing perception that in certain cases it may be preferable to participate actively in treatment rather than be passively medicated or operated upon. Such alternative approaches to health, as well as exercise and nutritional measures or development of a preventive life-style, are quite similar to the implicit goals of chi gong. The benefits of noninvasive treatment and natural methods, especially in chronic illness or in nonorganic diseases, are gaining attention.

Twenty years ago TCM, Western medicine, and the specializations of each ruled their separate domains, viewing the others with contempt and envy, and the patient lost out. The combined treatment recently attempted in China might be implemented in appropriate ways worldwide. The idea of combining treatments to achieve high effectiveness plainly has merit. Since in most cases no single medical technique can cover the entire scope of disease, the ideal practice would be to abandon preconceived notions, use the strong points of one treatment to make up for the weaknesses of another, and let the therapeutic approaches work together in harmony and synergy.

Since mainland China has begun opening up, many people from all over the world have traveled to China for medical treatment. They come for Chinese medicine and acupuncture after the treatments available in their own countries prove ineffective. In recent years a flurry of patients have visited China for chi gong treatment. The patients who have benefited from chi gong medical treatment include Paul Dong, who summarizes his experience:

Ten years ago, I was afflicted with many chronic diseases, including constipation, insomnia, aching all over my head, and dizziness caused by Ménière's disease. In 1980, I decided to vacation in China to visit my relatives and also to go for treatment from an acupuncturist in Shanghai. After my treatment was begun, I told him that I could only stay a few days. He became quite serious and said: "I will be honest with you since you are my friend. I cannot cure your chronic illness other than by giving you one or two months of treatment since you have to come back every other day for at least thirty to forty times." He advised that I take the opportunity to learn chi gong and cure myself through regular practice.

He introduced me to Ms. Tian Wen-yang, a chi gong master, who taught me the "quiet style" (described in chapter 8). It took her only a few hours every day for three days to see to it that I did everything correctly; she emphasized that I do it every day, in a natural and relaxed way, while keeping a clear and happy mind. Subsequently, I had the opportunity to learn Standing-on-Stake from Master Yu Yong-nian in Beijing (see chapter 7).

After returning to America, I kept practicing chi gong continuously for one year, and the four health problems described above were cured without the use of any other medical intervention. With regard to my chronic constipation, I had previously visited three medical and surgical specialists. One suggested an operation which would have cost me up to four thousand dollars. Learning chi gong cost me no more than fifty dollars. As for my headaches, had I taken the doctor's suggested course of testing and treatment, it would have cost another two thousand dollars. By performing chi gong exercises as the medical treatment, I recovered from this sickness at the same time, as well as from Ménière's disease! Even if one suffers from several different diseases, chi gong could possibly prove effective for all, because the condition of the whole body is improved.

Most of the people of mainland China have low incomes. They can barely scrape by, and it's almost beyond their means to go to the doctor. Not only does chi gong treat sickness and relieve their pain, but also their financial plight.

Chi gong is no panacea, and not everyone is affected positively. But, in general, it can serve as one of the techniques for treating a disease, and its effects are satisfactory. The rise of the chi gong clinic is in line with the needs and the trend of the times. At the time when the chi gong clinics were becoming popular, Dong toured the interiors of several in Guangzhou and Beijing. Besides the chi gong expert, a table and chairs, and some charts on the walls, no medical instruments of any kind, no nurses, and no medicine dispensaries were seen. The chi gong expert relies on nothing but his or her own hands to provide treatment for the sitting and recuperating patient. Each patient is examined every day or every other day, and chronic patients are taught chi gong exercises that they can do at home to augment the effect of the treatment initiated by the application of external chi.

In recent years, chi gong clinics on a somewhat larger scale, equipped with modern instruments and nursing staff have been established. There are reportedly six clinics on the grandest scale, one in every major metropolitan area. The largest of these, Bei Dai He Qi Gong Clinic, is located in Hebei province, 398 kilometers from Beijing, a five-hour-and-forty-five-minute trip by train. It is furnished with three hundred beds and staffed with forty chi gong experts and nurses. The nurses are all practitioners of chi gong. This facility serves three functions, including chi gong research, chi gong teaching, and clinical treatment. The building, whose construction was funded by the central government, is two stories high and covers an extensive area. The entire facility has a staff of about a hundred. Since 1984, it has also put out a quarterly journal, China Qi Gong, with a circulation of about eighty thousand. Foreign medical personnel frequently come to tour the facility. The patients admitted to the facility are all high-ranking officials. In recent years, in connection with the government's policy of opening up the country to foreigners, applications are also being accepted from foreign patients.

Bei Dai He is famous throughout northern China as a favorite resort area, tourist destination, and summer getaway. Situated by the seashore on the southern flank of the city of Qin Huang Dao, it has about ten kilometers of shore line, mild breezes, beautiful scenery, and a quiet, charming environment. In addition, it has extensive hot springs bathing areas. Before the People's Republic of China was established, English, American, and Japanese businessmen, diplomats, and wealthy people built retreats and established long-term residences here. The climate never becomes severely cold or unbearably hot, and from May to October each year, large numbers of tourists pour in. The greatest influx takes place during the summer, when people come to bathe in the ocean.

Bei Dai He Qi Gong Clinic was not built because of the recent popularity of chi gong, however. It was built in 1956, and, when the ills of many high-ranking officials were cured at the facility over the years, the government decided to invest heavily in an expansion of the site. Because of the facility's outstanding staff and the excellent use of both TCM and Western medicine, the cure rate is very high and the clinic enjoys the finest reputation. Mr. Zhao Bo Feng is the head of the facility. He is associate editor of *China Qi Gong*, and his published works include *One Hundred Questions about Qi Gong Therapy*. In the work's seventy-first question, Can Qi Gong Cure Cancer?, he states:

> Cancer constantly attracts the attention of the medical community and is taken seriously by people, and accordingly the human effort and financial resources expended on cancer research all over the world are increasing rapidly every year. As a result, the number of techniques for cancer treatment are also constantly increasing. All of these techniques, however, require one of the following two features: clearing out the locus of the cancerous growth, with such methods as surgery and radiation therapy, or changing the internal environment of the body to increase its resistance, with Chinese "out-with-the-bad" and "in-with-the-good" medicine and immunotherapy. In the early stages of cancer, some people

can recover through these treatments, but in the middle and late stages their effectiveness is less than ideal. The question of whether qi gong therapy can cure cancer is a matter of great interest to the many victims of the disease. Considering the mechanism of qi gong as a medical treatment, it can indeed change the internal environment of the body, improve the constitution, and strengthen the body's resistance and immune system, coinciding with the second required feature for any cancer treatment. Thus, quite a few patients use qi gong as an additional treatment at the same time when they use the techniques of surgery, chemotherapy, radiation therapy, or Chinese medicine, and the clinical results have not been bad. Furthermore, in some individual cases, qi gong therapy has proved remarkably effective for some patients in the late stage of cancer in conditions where it would have been impossible to apply other techniques such as surgery. In some cases the cancerous growth shrank, in some cases the symptoms showed clear signs of improvement or disappeared, and quite a few people survived far longer than the doctors had predicted they could live. Therefore, it may be said that qi gong does indeed have a certain effect on cancer.[2]

Bei Da Hei Clinic is the model for China's use of chi gong therapy. The facility has a cure rate as high as 78 percent. For Western-type hospitals in China the cure rate was about 82 percent.[3] The clinic uses chi gong as the main treatment, and TCM, especially acupuncture and massage, as well as Western medicine when needed. The uses of chi gong, as elsewhere, include the patients practicing chi gong themselves and the supplemental application of external chi treatment. Different kinds of chi gong are used for different diseases. Other criteria for selecting the chi gong treatment include the age and physical condition of the patient, and the stage of the disease.

Notes

1. See, for example, Cui Lili, "Fitness and Health Through Chi Gong," *Beijing Review,* 24–30 April 1989.

2. Zhao Bo Feng, *One Hundred Questions about Qi Gong Therapy* (Gansu: Gansu Publishing Company, 1984), p. 62.

3. Edgar Snow, *Red China Today* (New York: Random House, 1970), 304.

5

How Chi Gong Works on Cancer

Haughtiness invites ruin; humility receives benefits.

—I Ching (*The Book of Changes*)

Paul Dong has a personal interest in the effect of chi gong on cancer which he explains as follows:

> Because several of my relatives and friends died of cancer, I always felt particularly fearful of cancer. When I came across a Chinese book on five chi gong exercise techniques and discovered that chi gong can cure cancer, I became highly interested and started collecting materials on this subject. I also went to China in 1984 to see for myself, and found that it is definitely true that chi gong is being used to cure cancer. In the eleven years since 1979, the Chinese have cured hundreds of cancer victims through chi gong, and thousands upon thousands have used chi gong to achieve improvement and to prolong their lives. When news of this spread outside China, many medical professionals from other countries came to mainland China to observe. Members of the staff at Harvard Medical School have shown great interest in this area and have been to China twice to observe the practice. According to the article "Cancer Does Not Mean Death" by Ke Yan,[1] an American oncologist (the article doesn't give the doctor's name) visited China and requested an interview with the pioneer of chi gong cancer treatment, Mrs. Guo Lin (1906–1984). Guo Lin said, "Even if I tell you about it, you wouldn't believe me. You'd better

85

find a patient of mine to talk to." The oncologist found quite a few of her patients in the Beijing district chi gong cancer class, spent four days talking with them, and saw the facts for himself.

Doctors have taken two contrasting approaches to cancer. The first approach is to consider the cancer to be an isolated condition localized at one spot in the body and to attack it directly using chemicals, surgery, or radiation. The second approach, which is gaining more and more prominence today, is to consider the condition of the whole person as the environment for the cancer, and to strengthen the body's resistance to cancer. This may come under the modern heading of psychoneuroimmunology (discussed in chapter 13) and relies on many factors, including exercise, diet, and mental imaging to combat the disease. Chi gong is part of this second approach.

The use of chi gong cancer treatment in China originated with Ms. Guo Lin, a Chinese traditional painter, mentioned above. In 1949, she was afflicted with uterine cancer and had it removed by surgery in Shanghai. The cancer recurred in 1960. This time it had metastasized to the bladder, and she had another operation in Beijing to remove part of the bladder that was cancerous. When she had another relapse, the doctors gave her six months to live. However, she did not give up hope, and in her struggle against cancer, she remembered that her grandfather, a Taoist priest, had taught her as a child to practice chi gong. She determinedly began to research and practice chi gong, hoping to recover her health in this way. After initial practice with no effect, she turned to the ancient chi gong texts willed to her by her grandfather and created her own exercise schedule. She practiced diligently for two hours every day, and in half a year her cancer subsided. She was strongly convinced of chi gong's ability to cure diseases, and in 1970 started giving lessons in what she called New Chi Gong Therapy. According to Cyrus Lee, Master

Guo's therapy is not based on the external energy (*wei* chi) of others, but upon the inner energy (*nei* chi) of the patient (for these distinctions, review chapter 1, "Special Section on Chi"). Her therapy combines "active and passive exercises in three stages: relaxation (*sung jing*), concentration (*yi lian*), and breathing (*tiao hsi*)."[2]

By 1977 Master Guo had achieved spectacular results and proclaimed publicly that chi gong can cure cancer. Cancer victims from all over immediately streamed into Beijing to take part in the chi gong cancer therapy class she had organized. Each day three hundred to four hundred people studied chi gong techniques for cancer treatment with her. Until her death in 1984 she worked tirelessly, curing hundreds of cancer patients, while easing the pain and prolonging the lives of thousands more. Mrs. Wong Chung-siu, a student of Guo Lin's currently living in Fremont, California, told Paul Dong that Guo Lin's pinnacle of success came in 1982. Aided by nine assistants she had trained, Guo Lin held nine cancer classes of seventy students each, meeting three times a day. With her nine assistants to help her, she was able over the next two years to travel all over China to twenty provincial capitals to teach and lecture at the request of many local health care and medical departments, and she became a national celebrity before her death in 1984 (twenty years after her life had been given up by Western medicine).

Because Guo Lin had demonstrated that her chi gong techniques were able to cure cancer, people trained in other styles of chi gong were eager to see if they could achieve the same results. Among these other styles, quiet gong and movement gong also demonstrated the same ability to achieve cures or alleviation of cancer. Paul Dong judges from the Chinese literature that movement gong is more effective in curing cancer. The technique used by Guo Lin combines both movement chi gong and meditation chi gong (movement first and quiet gong afterward).

One type of movement gong is Flying Crane, which is quite

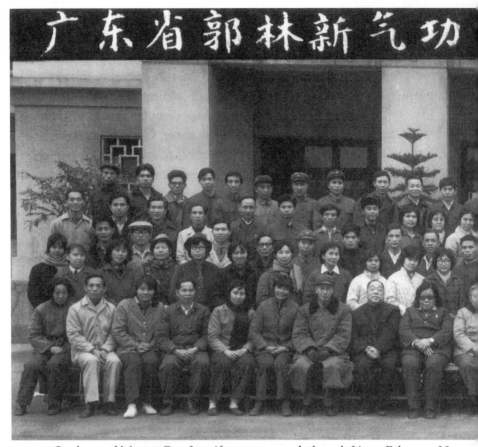

Students of Master Guo Lin (front row, ninth from left) on February 28, 1981, in Guangzhou. (*Photo courtesy of Ms. Wong Chung-siu.*)

popular in mainland China. According to reports, it has cured many cancer patients. In a journal *Qi Gong of the Flying Crane,* published in Beijing, an article "Fight Cancer with the True Qi," written by Xie Hua,[3] states that the Beijing Flying Crane Club invited eleven cancer victims to participate in an experiment. After three months of practicing chi gong, they showed varying degrees of improvement. Among them, Li Shan-cheng showed the most notable effects. Li, fifty-nine years old at the time, had cancer of the esophagus and was

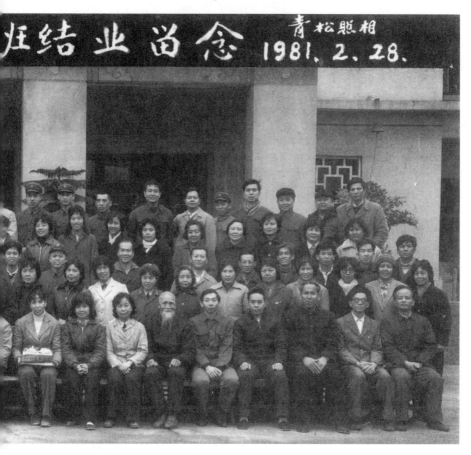

结业留念 青松照相 1981. 2. 28.

unable to eat; in fact, he couldn't even swallow water. He was emaciated. Then he watched a report on TV about chi gong curing cancer and joined a Flying Crane therapy class. After practicing chi gong for ten days, he had a check-up and discovered that his tumor had become smaller, and he was able to eat again. With this encouragement, he practiced chi gong an hour at a time, four times a day. After three months, he had made a complete recovery and went back to work as usual. He credited chi gong with saving his life.

In Hebei province's Tianjin University, the chi gong class for the fourth quarter of 1983 included fifteen cancer victims (the categories

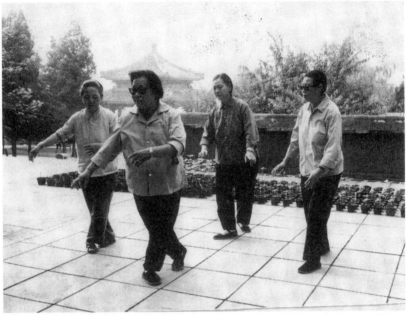

Master Guo demonstrates her chi gong for patients. (*Photo courtesy of Ms. Wong Chung-siu.*)

were cancer of the liver, the stomach, the mammary gland, and the rectum). After six months to a year of practicing chi gong, not one of them had died. Their conditions showed various levels of improvement, and all of the patients experienced the triple benefit of eating, sleeping, and feeling well. They were also firm in their conviction that "to exercise right is to survive." The styles of chi gong that they practiced were Standing-On-Stake and meditation gong, which will be described in chapters 8 and 12 respectively.

All kinds of cases regarding the cure of cancer with different styles of chi gong are frequently reported in chi gong magazines. The conclusion may be that no matter what chi gong style is used, it is possible to cure cancer. The simple truth is that every style of chi gong adheres to three principles: (*a*) achieving a state of tranquility, (*b*) relaxation and release of tension, (*c*) commitment and develop-

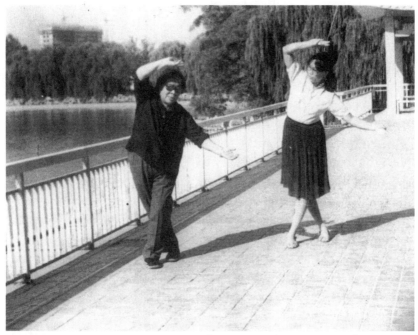

Master Guo instructing Ms. Wong Chung-siu. (*Photo courtesy of Ms. Wong Chung-siu.*)

ment of willpower. And each of these principles is important in one's fight against cancer. In addition, we think that the reason Guo Lin's chi gong was especially effective is because she had her patients train in groups. Group practice is the best way to arouse interest and bring good cheer. Interest helps one concentrate on doing the chi gong exercises, and cheerfulness produces a beneficial effect on the organism. As the first step in curing cancer, Guo Lin had the patients come together as a group and swear an oath to resist cancer, for the purpose of increasing their fighting spirit. Willpower was applied as a healing technique. In a large group of patients (Guo Lin's cancer therapy groups usually consisted of seventy people), there would be one or two of a more sensitive disposition, achieving the beneficial effects of chi gong earlier than the others. As soon as one or two patients had shown good results, the rest of the patients would be encouraged to have greater confidence, and as we know, a positive attitude plays a role in curing disease. Also, if people practice chi gong exercises alone and then fail to achieve results, they are more likely to become discouraged.

One reason for the negative impact of failure acknowledged in Western medicine is that the feeling of helplessness appears to suppress the immune system's ability to resist tumor development.[4] On the other hand, fostering positive images appears to strengthen immunological competence.[5] Lawrence Leshan has pointed to psychological factors in cancer causation since the fifties.[6] Specific methods to fight cancer successfully with visualization techniques were introduced in the U.S. by Carl Simonton, M.D., in the early seventies.[7] Thus there are reasons to think that a positive attitude improves and negative thoughts decrease the immune mechanism's ability to defend the body.

Much, but not all of chi gong's effect is based on entering a state of meditation. In meditation, there are no distractions, depressing thoughts, or worries. The body's functions are able to return to normal by relaxation, which is the key to balancing the circulation of the chi and the blood. In Chinese traditional medical theory, stimulating the circulation of the chi and blood is the main healing method. Additionally, a sense of happiness is achieved in meditation, and that is a major wellspring of increased confidence and fighting spirit.

The several effects described above are important mechanisms for treating any disease. As the term psychoneuroimmunology implies, these mechanisms include both psychological and physiological elements. As we know, the psychological and the physiological aspects operate in interdependent ways. From the physiological point of view, the Shanghai Institute of Medical Science's Institute for the Combined Use of Chinese and Western Medicine has conducted a study

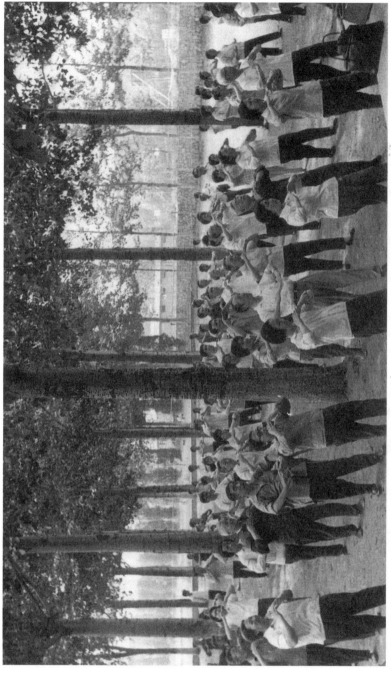

A Guo Lin patient group exercise in Beijing. (*Photo courtesy of China Sports*)

on the effects of chi gong and *tai ji chuan* on elderly people's endocrine systems (the pituitary, thyroid, and sex glands). They invited forty-seven elderly people of the same age, sixty-six years old, to perform chi gong exercises regularly. After doing this for several weeks, the capabilities of their pituitary, thyroid, and sex glands were shown to have increased. This strengthening and stabilizing of the endocrine system can have a beneficial regulating effect on the vigor of the whole body's metabolism.

This is not to suggest that we understand the extent of chi gong's effects on cancer. We do know that practicing chi gong exercises influences many of the body's mechanisms. For instance, it not only raises the capabilities of the endocrine system, it also has a regulating effect on cyclic adenosine monophosphate (cAMP) and cyclic guanosine monophosphate (cGMP). These two substances play a vital bioenergetic role in phosphorylation, which is the key to respiration and thus the oxygen provision for all of the body's cells. As we will review below, oxygen prevents cancer growth. In addition, cyclic AMP is familiar as an intracellular signal transforming stimuli from outside the cell into a response by the cell, and therefore could play an important role in our immune system.

In a recent study, Wang Chong-xing and collaborators at the Shanghai Institute of Hypertension reported at a world conference on chi gong on improvement in the ratio of cAMP/cGMP within one year of chi gong practice.[8] It is claimed that the concentration and physiological stability (expressed in a stable ratio) of these two enzyme messengers play major roles in the normal regulation and maintenance of health. It is assumed that cancer cells thrive when the blood cAMP content is low. Ding Shen and other investigators, reporting at the same world conference, have found that the practice of chi gong, among other beneficial effects, increases the cAMP content of the blood which may explain part of chi gong's effect on cancer.

Another important factor in cancer growth is whether or not the body's oxygen content is sufficient. Beijing's Qi Gong and Cancer Research Unit has conducted many experiments on this aspect. When the body is deficient in oxygen, cancer cells grow; and when the body is rich in oxygen, cancer cells die. One explanation for the sense of serenity produced by entering a state of deep meditation through chi gong is the increase in the absorption of oxygen. In ancient China, Taoist priests chose to meditate underneath the pine tree because they had discovered that the pine exudes the greatest amount of oxygen.

The above points are possible explanations by modern science of several mechanisms by which chi gong cures cancer. From the point of view of Chinese traditional medicine, chi gong has the functions of activating the body's vital forces (chi), strengthening the blood's circulation, balancing the *yin* and the *yang*, stimulating the conductivity of the meridians and improving the psychological state. Chinese medical theory emphasizes that chi is the driving force of life. The body's health is determined by the strength or weakness of its chi. As soon as the chi is weakened, the "blood is clogged," the *yin* and *yang* lose their balance, and disease will result. Research by the Bei Dai He Chi Gong Clinic indicates that after doing a chi gong exercise for a certain period of time (we judge this to be approximately forty minutes), the body's internal regional blood volume increases by 30 percent and the body temperature rises two to three degrees Celsius. For the Chinese, these facts demonstrate the way that chi gong acts to clear the meridians—unclog the blood—and moderate the chi and blood. In other words, when the chi and the blood are flowing freely, the body will maintain physiological balance (the balance of *yin* and *yang*), and diseases will disappear of themselves.

In recent years, scientists and medical specialists have been turning their attention to the immune system for the purpose of fighting disease. China took up this point more than two thousand years ago. As *The Emperor's Classic* states in "Questions and Answers": "Be imperturbable and the true chi will come to you; concentrate the inner spirit and well-being follows." This signifies that if the body's energy is at its full level, it will not sicken. Chi gong exercises bring out and mobilize the body's latent strength, raise the body's energy level, and activate the cells of the immune system, causing a feeling of well-being.

Many studies have demonstrated that people suffering from emotional damage, tension, a low level of energy, depression, and irritability have a markedly higher rate of cancer occurrence. Through the practice of chi gong, especially when reaching the level of the deep meditative state, a whole set of beneficial psychological and spiritual conditions emerge, including emotional well-being, spiritual happiness, stability of mood, and complete relaxation of the body. This directly inspires the patient's confidence of defeating cancer, as well as benefiting the body's dynamic balance, and as a consequence makes a positive contribution to the healing and comfort of the body.

Besides one's own practice of chi gong, another method of treating cancer is through the use of a chi gong expert who can provide relief by transmitting external chi from his body to that of the patient, thereby purportedly killing cancer cells. Dr. Feng Li-da, vice-president, General Hospital of the Chinese Navy, Beijing, and professor of immunology, Beijing College of Traditional Chinese Medicine, has done many experiments in this area. She reported that by transmitting external chi for one minute, a chi gong expert can destroy 90 percent of colon and dysentery bacilli, and in ten minutes 60 percent of a flu virus. In sixty minutes, the rate of destroyed uterine cancer cells is also around 60 percent, and that of destroyed gastric cancer cells 25 percent. A twenty-gram tumor on a mouse disappeared within a five-week period of external chi treatment. A few of the experiments referred to above were reported in the following press release of November 28, 1983, by the New China (Xinhua) News Agency:

A meeting for the evaluation and demonstration of the action of chi gong on certain bacteria has recently been held, presided over by Feng, Li Da, deputy superintendent of the Navy General Hospital and director of the Immunology Research Division.

Test tubes filled respectively with coliform bacillus and dysentery bacteria, golden and white staphylococcus, and virus were handed over one by one to a chi gong master, who held each of the tubes firmly in his hand for a minute to release external energy (chi) at it. A projector displayed the image of each experimental sample on a screen. Under an electronic microscope, the bacteria were shown to be expanding, cracking, and dissolving, being killed by chi gong.

From the immunological standpoint, Feng has thus demonstrated that chi energy is an objective reality. Furthermore, she has confirmed that chi gong is effective to a certain degree in treating B-hepatitis. There is also encouraging preliminary evidence of the therapeutic effect of chi gong with respect to the treatment of guinea pigs suffering from ascites (an accumulation of fluid in the abdomen) caused by cancer.

Dr. Feng declared that in mainland China chi gong has now advanced from the prescientific phase to a new epoch in which modern scientific methods are employed in its study. The study of chi gong has been conducive to the development of immunology and other sciences.

Another example: A Japanese cancer victim, Ansei Shonin, who had a tumor in the lower part of his head, deeply imbedded in his nasal cavity, made a special trip from Japan to Beijing's General Hospital of the People's Liberation Army to undergo external chi treatment. A chi gong expert performed twelve days of external chi treatment, and as a result Ansei Shonin's tumor, as large as an egg, shrunk, and his pain was also distinctly eased.

Why external chi works toward strengthening of the cells and the immune responses of the body in the case of healing a disease, and appears to kill or otherwise interrupt and reverse the growth of cells (or bacteria) in the case of cancer (or the influencing of bacterial cultures) is not known. To the best of our knowledge, it is due to the different intent of the qi gong master. This may be similar to visualization or imaging therapy, as applied in Western alternative medical approaches. As part of the therapy, the determination is made in advance whether the patient will visualize growth of healthy or destruction of cancerous cells in his or her own body.

In conclusion, then, cancer victims apparently can achieve effective treatment by practicing chi gong as shown by Master Guo. But one might suggest that if the patient is too weak or for other reasons unable to practice chi gong regularly and vigorously, external chi should be tried as a cure or used as a supplement to chi gong. Finally, as described in the previous chapter regarding practices in the Bei Da Hei Clinic, combinations of "internal" and "external" chi with dietetic therapy and Western medical science may all be attempted when looking for a cure for cancer.

Notes

1. Ke Yan, "Cancer Does Not Mean Death," *Beijing Literature*, July 1982, 43.

2. Cyrus Lee, "Qi Gong (Breath Exercise) and Its Major Models," *Chinese Culture* 24 (September 1984): 71–79. The description was quoted by Prof. Lee from Guo Lin's book *Hsin Qigong Liao Fa* (Hofei: Science and Technology Press, 1980), 4.

3. Xie Hua, "Fight Cancer with the True Qi," *Qi Gong of the Flying Crane*, Beijing, n.d.

4. See for example, M. Visintainer et al. in *Science* 216 (1982): 437–40.

5. See for example, P. Lansky in *Perspectives in Biology and Medicine* 23 (1982): 496–503.

6. See for example, Lawrence Leshan, *You Can Fight for Your Life: Emotional Factors in the Causation of Cancer* (New York: Evans, 1977).

7. O. C. Simonton et al., *Getting Well Again* (Los Angeles: J. P. Tarcher, 1978).

8. Wang Chong-xing et al. in *First World Conference for Academic Exchange of Medical Qi Gong*, 1988, 85.

6

Empty Force -
The Mystery of Chi

Mastering others requires power;
Mastering oneself needs strength.

—Lao Tzu, *Tao Te Ching*, 33

There are many varieties of chi gong, as many as thirty-three hundred according to Gao He-ting, president of the Beijing College of Traditional Chinese Medicine. Over time, different schools have developed separate styles of skills and practice. Empty Force is just one of these, but it is used especially to develop skills in healing and the martial arts, in particular the ability to affect another person without physical contact. Because it is one of the most powerful methods (and also difficult to master) one should not engage in it without the personal guidance of a chi gong master. We will therefore not provide descriptions of the exercise, but use a discussion of Empty Force as a background to manifestations of external chi beyond the healing context.

The practice of Empty Force relies on a strictly internal martial art, whereby the mind and the intention of the practitioner deliver the action. Empty Force produces high energy very rapidly. No sooner has the thought occurred than the force may reach the object.

For instance, lifting the hand can throw another person to the ground. Thus, a chi gong practitioner must learn through conscious will to exercise control over the consequences of his or her actions so that no life is threatened. But when there is a surprise attack from an adversary there may be no time to exercise conscious control, and if in such cases the assault is perceived as a threat to life, expert activation of Empty Force is almost certain to result in the death of the attacker. Because of these aspects the Chinese describe this transmittal of energy without physical contact through space by thought as *Lin* (powerful) *Kung* (empty) *Jing* (strength). The traditional English translation is Empty Force.

Paul Dong has personally become acquainted with Empty Force masters; foremost among these was Yu Peng-si (1902–1983). According to one of Yu's students, the martial arts master Wong Docfai, there are two kinds of thought, the good and the bad. Good thought can adjust the *yin* and *yang* within one's body to restore equilibrium and maintain good health, as well as produce a therapeutic effect on a sick person. Bad thought can hurt another person by producing physiological changes, headache, dizziness, nausea, even death.

Master Yu was a medical doctor trained in Germany, who taught at Shango University in Shanghai while giving chi gong training in his spare time at home. As a young man he learned martial arts from Wang Xiang-ji, a famous martial arts master. Later, Master Yu went to Tibet to learn Tibetan Buddhist meditation. Subsequently, while living in Shanghai he came to know Le Wan-zhi, a professor at Ji Tang University, from whom he learned the Empty Force method. By combining and improving the three different chi gong styles he had trained in, he ultimately developed the Yu-style Empty Force technique. One has to practice a minimum of three hours a day for three years before one can exercise its enormous strength. Master Yu became a legend and trained many students. According to columnist

Huang Shi-chi of the *Centre Daily News* in Hong Kong, he was told by one of Yu's closest friends, Brother Su, of the marvels of his technique. The students practiced Empty Force standing ten to thirty feet apart, and raised their hands to launch attacks on each other. Those who were weak had to keep retreating or would otherwise be thrown to the ground. Yu's own power was such that with a wave of his hand he could force his students to leap back or be thrown tens of feet. They might also be tossed into the air or made to turn somersaults repeatedly before falling to the ground. When Yu pointed his fingers downward while exerting pressure from a distance, students on the ground would be unable to get up, regardless of how hard they tried. Only when Yu would lift his hand would the students be able to rise again. Brother Su related to Huang Shi-chi:

> Once I was chatting with Yu in a room while some of his students were practicing in the open yard outside and others were taking a rest. On the spur of the moment Yu said: "Watch, I am going to shoot Empty Force at them." As he began his concentration, all the students, including those at rest, were forced to retreat from the house. It was indeed more marvelous than what one would read in *wuxia* (martial arts) novels.

At the invitation of Professor Martin Lee of Stanford University in Palo Alto, California, Master Yu came to the United States in 1981. One of his students, Xia Chang-fang, lost no time inviting Yu to stay in his house and organized a chi gong training class for him. Subsequently, the San Francisco martial arts community became involved in learning Empty Force, and there originated an intense debate on whether Empty Force was a legitimate phenomenon or a deception. In the West Coast magazine *Inside Kung Fu* a letter to the editor stated that Empty Force was not to be believed. To gain firsthand experience, Paul Dong contacted Master Yu and his wife

Min Ou-yang who told him: "The only way to ascertain whether Empty Force is real and how the power is produced is to learn it. You'll get to the bottom of it if you persist in practicing for three years." One of the students was Jane Hallander, a reporter who wrote a special article on Empty Force in the magazine *Karate Kung Fu.* [1] The Research Association of Chinese Qi Gong Health Exercises has held demonstrations by Wong Doc-fai, who as Yu's student recruited Jane Hallander. As far as Dong knows, in the Bay area the other top students of Yu are Xia Chang-fang and Master X, who asked not to be identified.

Of these masters in the Yu-style Empty Force technique, Xia appears the most seasoned. At one time he taught *tai ji quan* (see chapter 11) in Berkeley, where he is now teaching at a high school. From childhood he had been a martial arts fan and learned *tai ji* and *Ren Yi* Fist, a top martial art. He has been traveling in quest of famous masters to improve his skills. He learned Empty Force from Yu Peng-si whom he asked during his stay in Palo Alto to organize a class in the Fort Mason District of San Francisco. At that time he was introduced to Cai Song-fang, an expert in *Wujishi Chio Gong* (Unlimited Force) from Canton, whom he took as a teacher. By combining the skills of Masters Yu and Cai, after years of hard practice, Xia now has become a top master of Empty Force.

One day when Xia visited Hong Kong, his friends (including columnist Huang Shi-chi mentioned earlier) held a dinner party in his honor. After the dinner he was asked to give a demonstration. With just a slight wave of his hand he made Mr. Mai, a guest standing ten feet away, retreat five or six paces. There was a stone pillar in the hall and Mr. Mai was asked to stand behind it. Then Xia released his energy and despite the protection of the pillar, Mr. Mai staggered back and nearly fell to the ground. Then Huang saw the opportunity and asked Xia to inject energy into him. The two of them stood face-to-face, separated by a distance of about a foot. Xia placed his hands on the wrists of Huang who reported that he felt the chi flow through his body. Since Huang is a chi gong practitioner, he knew how to utilize and absorb the energy.

Here are some of Paul Dong's personal experiences with Empty Force:

I told you something about Master Yu; now I want to talk about Xia's other teacher. Cai was a native of Shanghai, presently living in Canton, who came to San Francisco at the invitation of Xia and the local martial arts community. Cai gave a demonstration at which my student Paul Wong was present. Cai asked the students to push him, and each tried it in turn, but the master was immovable. "What was more amazing," said Paul Wong, "his eyes looked strange, staring at a point three feet away. The student who tried to push him had to fall back three feet. When Cai shifted his gaze to about seven feet away, the student had to fall back more! Then another student tried to help him but was unable to hold him up; instead they both had to retreat together!"

A similar account of Master Cai was rendered by Dr. Ho Zhong-Xian, a practitioner of Chinese traditional medicine, who came to the U.S. from Canton in 1980. I asked him whether he knew Cai Song-fang. He said that he had often seen him teaching in a public park and that Cai was most adept at flying a kite. "What is that," I asked him. He explained with a smile: "That is the art of forcing back people like paper birds blown by a gust of wind to more than thirty feet away." He added, "It is impossible for anyone to push him, but for him to push you back or down all he needs is to use his eyes and perhaps his thought."

When Master Cai was in the Bay area I joined his classes for two months. We practiced twice a week with several of my friends. Once, when I asked him to show me his chi, he told me to put up my hands with the palms facing the sky. He then sent chi into my palms which became hot. When I asked him to fly me "like a kite" he explained that this could be done only with experienced students; others would get hurt. I asked such an experienced student, Sandy Rosenberg, a Ph.D. from the University of California, what he felt when Master Cai did this to him. He said that it was hard to explain, but "when I receive the chi I feel something strange and I have to get away from it." The sensation of electromagnetic fields is not a common experience; Sandy acquired his ability to feel it through chi gong training. Chi is like a magnetic field which people normally do not feel, but that could hurt you nonetheless. This is the explanation of the known dangers of experimenting with chi forces if you have not had any training. But once you have been trained and are sensitive to the field, you will recognize the danger and get away from it. If you are inexperienced you might not fly like a kite, but become injured instead.

Empty Force and Unlimited Force have equal power and both use the eyes to direct the thought to throw people to the ground. Which is superior? All I know is that Empty Force was invented fifty years ago while Unlimited Force was a secret skill practiced by the Palace Guards of ancient China. Cai acquired it through some secret channel.

Before the death of Yu Peng-si, who lived in Shanghai, Cai lived in Canton. So there was a master in the North and a master in the South. Both had their teachers. Among those who taught Yu were Wang Siang-zai and Le Wan-zhi. Master Wang once beat a Japanese judo and sword expert with his stick. The story goes as follows:

In 1939, upon hearing about the superior skills of Wang, a Japanese colonel named Sawai made a special trip to Peking to see him. First he tried judo, but Wang responded with flying him away. Then, assuming Wang knew nothing about swordsmanship, Sawai attacked with his sword while Wang wielded a stick. Immediately at the start of their engagement, Sawai was tossed up into the air, sword and all, and then fell to the ground. Wang had merely lifted his stick. Stunned and subdued Sawai knelt before Wang and besought his instructions.

In the *Orthodox Yi Fist*, a general magazine published in Hong Kong, one of Wang's disciples related the following story:

A middle-weight boxing champion from Italy came to Peking as a tourist and upon being told that there was a famous martial arts master, called at Wang's residence and asked for a match. As the boxer threw his first punch at the master, Wang, instead of warding the fist off, merely gave it a pinch, thereby throwing him to the ground. Astounded, the champion thought it was magic and, not daring to try again, acknowledged defeat.

About Yu's other tutor, Le Wan-zhi, another story is told. Once he forewarned a student that he would deliver Empty Force over the phone. The student, not wanting to appear irreverent, but secretly not believing such power, called Master Le the next day. To his great surprise, upon hearing Le's voice, he felt pulled to the ground and had to continue his call in prone position!

Le's pupil Wang Yeh-jing reported in *Panorama Monthly*, published in Hong Kong: One day during World War II, when Shanghai was under Japanese occupation, a Chinese woman was being insulted in the street by four Japanese soldiers, but nobody dared to intervene. Master Le happened to pass by and he sent out his Empty Force at the four soldiers, seriously injuring them; reportedly one died of the injuries received. It was whispered around Shanghai that only Le was capable of performing this magic. But when Le was queried by Wang, he denied it as his doing, but said, "The Japanese soldiers who insulted this woman were surely a bad lot; anyone who killed them is a patriot, whoever it may be."

Before the Communist takeover, a group of foreigners in Shanghai, eager to witness Empty Force for themselves, paid Master Le a visit. Le offered them a demonstration of a made-up game, Preventing Someone from Entering a Door. He challenged them to enter his home and promised to pay anyone successful twenty yuan, equivalent to two hundred dollars in present money. Needless to say, nobody won that bet!

Although I have no proof to substantiate the game of Preventing Someone from Entering a Door, the story cannot be without foundation, because there is indirect evidence. The skill of Master Feng Xia-zho, currently teaching Empty Force at Berkeley, is a case in point. I made an appointment to meet him in a Berkeley restaurant. At forty, with his ruddy complexion and a light, yet forceful gait, Feng gives the impression of a man of unusual skill. I asked him many questions and then arranged to see him teaching his students at the gym in the evening. I arrived at 8 P.M. and all the students were there already, both male and female, four-fifths American. At my request Feng gave a demonstration of Empty Force by holding a chair in his hand, saying, "I am sending my force to the front of this chair and none of the students will be able to touch it." He then asked one of his students to run toward the chair. A psychology student from the University of California, Berkeley, dashed toward the chair but stopped a few inches short of it, unable to move any further. Instead he was forced to move back, panting heavily. I asked him later what made him pant. He said: "I began to feel short of breath on receiving the energy from Master Feng." Feng himself told me that by linking his chi to that of the student, he brought him under control. Once, he said, he inadvertently caused chest pain in someone who happened to be watching a demonstration Feng gave. The injured person needed to be treated by Feng, but recovered completely.

Feng also had a commercial shown on the West Coast Channel 26, in which he was surrounded by a number of husky men, who had to pull back in all directions as soon as Feng started to move. It was Chinese language TV. If it had been seen on American TV, it would almost certainly have been condemned as hype.

What we are talking about here is Empty Force. I know that it is not empty talk, because I have started training myself in this technique. However, I am told that out of every hundred persons who go in for this training only two or three will succeed, for the training is rigorous: three to four hours a day for at least three to five years. Who with a busy life-style in the U.S. will spare three hours a day?

Notes

1. Jane Hallander, "Sum-i: The Highest Stage of Martial Training," *Karate Kung Fu*, May 1986.

7

The Chi Gong Masters

Ch'i kung is a very sophisticated discipline in which one may spend a year, ten years, or a lifetime. But the benefits gained by its practitioners have kept it alive and developing for nearly four thousand years.

—Lily Siou, Ch'i Kung: The Art of Mastering the Unseen Life Force

According to chi gong master Zhao Jin-xiang, the ideal age to take up chi gong exercises is from fifteen to seventeen years old. Of course, he himself has often claimed that he began practicing chi gong at the age of five, but this is really too young for most individuals. Perhaps a child studying the piano could begin at the age of five to six, for if these five- to six-year-old children may not care much about practicing the piano at least the dexterity of their fingers can be trained. However, in chi gong that is not so. Chi gong requires entering the quiet state, the elimination of distracting thoughts, concentration, and relaxation, all of which are difficult for children to attain. Therefore, it is generally felt, and Paul Dong agrees, that the ideal age to begin chi gong training is between fifteen and seventeen years old.

The chi gong masters in China with a high level of power have practiced at least twenty years. If they have practiced chi gong from the age of fifteen, they would now be between thirty-five to forty years old. Those who are over forty will have practiced chi gong at least thirty years. The chi gong masters who have practiced for twenty to thirty years not only have abundant chi gong powers, they also have psychic powers (chapter 10 will discuss the relationship between chi gong and psychic powers). What follows are Dong's personal encounters with some of the most famous Chinese chi gong masters, but it is rumored in China that those with ultimate power do not reveal their talents. No one knows their names or whereabouts. Here follow Dong's personal opinions and observations.

Yu Yong-nian has been one of my most influential chi gong teachers. At present he is retired; formerly he was chairman of the Dentistry Department of Beijing Railroad General Hospital. From 1943 to the present he has practiced Standing-On-Stake chi gong. He is a disciple of China's famous martial arts specialist Wang Xiang-ji. Wang, a legendary figure in China in the 1930s, used Empty Force for attacking so that he could drive back his opponent without touching him. The Standing-On-Stake chi gong (discussed in chapter 8) was created by Wang and today there are about eight million people practicing this type of chi gong. It is an excellent way for preserving health and for self-healing, and it can certainly improve martial arts powers. Master Yu's writings include *A Way To Prolong Life*, published in February 1982 by Knowledge Publishers, Beijing. In the book, there is a detailed explanation of the meaning and the benefits of Standing-On-Stake. Master Yu explains that Master Wang had two kinds of disciples. One kind studied the art of attack and defense, and the other concentrated on preserving health. In his first year, Yu Yong-nian studied Standing-On-Stake for preserving health; later he studied Standing-On-Stake for the art of attack and defense. Thus, he is adept at both preserving health and the art of attack and defense. His Standing-On-Stake for maintaining health is very famous, but no one ever mentions his skill in the art of attack and defense. He is one of those people who do not reveal their talents. He doesn't show off his gifts except when necessary. At the chi gong conference in Xi'an in 1984, I saw a performance on stage in which two young people pushed him and couldn't make him move. I have been told that Master Yu's Empty Force is formidable.

Standing-On-Stake chi gong as taught by Master Yu can cure many diseases—for example, high blood pressure, heart disease, arthritis, lumbago, and paralysis induced by external injuries. The latter particularly catches people's attention. A writer, Ms. Fang Dian-zhen, suffered paralysis for many years and neither Chinese nor Western medicine could cure it. Later, she learned to practice Standing-On-Stake and recovered. She wrote an article, which was published in *China Qi Gong* 1, in 1984, which elicited several thousand letters from all over China.

When I was in Beijing in 1984 I spent two days with Master Yu to learn his chi gong techniques. The first day he took me to a park early in the morning to practice chi gong beside a lake with his group of students. He introduced me to a Ms. Peng who at age twenty-two still had not begun menstruating. She consulted Western trained doctors who could not help her. Then an instructor suggested she try chi gong. She joined Yu's morning class, and her menarche started after only three and a half months of practicing Standing-On-Stake.

During these two days I found Master Yu reluctant to talk about Empty Force other than mentioning that he was not particularly good at it, as compared to his teacher, Master Wang.

Four years later, Master Yu's student Lam Kam-Chuen came from England to visit me in Oakland. We discussed Master Yu's reluctance to talk about Empty Force and martial arts in particular. Lam gave me an insight when recounting that Master Yu had hidden Master Wang in his Beijing home during the time that the Gang of Four ruled the country and chi gong was considered politically subversive (see chapter 10). This may explain why many Chinese are afraid to talk to foreigners, as they are not sure whether the political climate may change again.

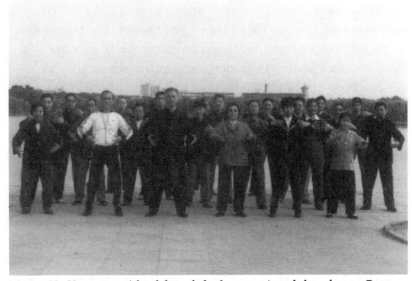

Master Yu Yong-nian (third from left, front row) with his class in Beijing, 1984. First from left is Ms. Peng; next to her is Paul Dong.

Tan Yao-qing of Guangxi Province and fifty years old as of this writing, is one of my chi gong teachers. He is the latest in a long line of herb doctors in his family, and he is an expert at chi gong for restoring and preserving. He has been written up hundreds of times in newspapers and in magazines in China.

In July 1985 I went to China to investigate chi gong on behalf of the Research Association of Chinese Qi Gong Exercise and the Center for Scientific Anomalies Research (CSAR), headed by Professor Marcello Truzzi of Eastern Michigan University. Wanting to meet Master Tan very much, I made an appointment to meet him in Guangzhou on September 27, 1985.

The next morning an audience of one hundred people, including Mr. Zhang and Mr. Wu, editor and reporter of the *Yang Cheng Evening News* respectively, were gathered at the People's Liberation Army Health Clinic. Eight female patients (between the ages of seventeen and twenty-five and from different hospitals) afflicted with

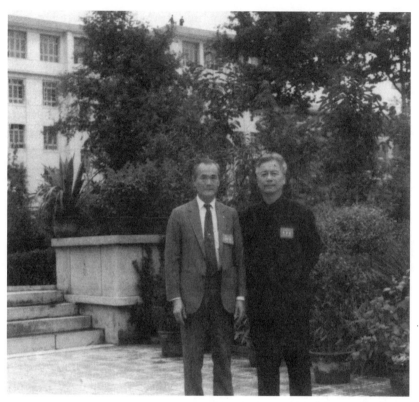

Paul Dong and Master Yu.

fibroadenoma[1] of the breast were given external chi by the master. Three claimed to have no more symptoms after one treatment, four were treated twice, and only one needed three treatments before she was free of symptoms. The hospital director and a female doctor, Wang Hong-yin, were present to verify that this treatment had removed their fibroadenomas. The news was published in the *Yang Cheng Evening News* on September 28, 1985.

Later, I heard from Wu Shi-gong, a reporter for the *Yang Cheng Evening News*, that Master Tan is best at healing fibroadenoma in women, with a 95 percent effectiveness rate. I asked him what the rate of effectiveness was for other illnesses, and he said there was some healing effect, but not very high, usually somewhere between 40 and 60 percent. I thought it was strange that his external chi was only effective on fibroadenoma, so I asked Master Tan why. He said he didn't know either. Perhaps it is because of the type of his external chi. In 1978 at the Shanghai Atomic Energy Research Institute, his external chi was tested and found to have infrared and magnetic effects; the magnetism had a strength of 1.25 gauss. As we said in chapter 1, the external chi produced by every chi gong master is different. Different types of external chi may cure different diseases. For example, the infrared chi is comparatively more effective for healing rheumatism.

Huang Ren-chong, one of my chi gong friends, was born in Shanghai and is forty-two years old as of this writing. He is now practicing chi gong professionally in the Shenzhen special economic zone in Guangdong Province. He practices Empty Force chi gong, and his force is quite substantial. He releases external chi from his palms. Because his external chi is so strong, it is very effective in curing diseases. He is called Demon-Palm Huang. There is a story describing how, in October of 1981, he healed a young woman with a bone fracture of the lumbar vertebra in Shanghai People's Liberation Army Hospital 765. Her bone fracture was the result of an unsuccessful suicide attempt in which she jumped from the third floor of a building. Her name was Cui Ping, and she had been a nurse in Xinyang City Advanced Hospital in Henan Province. She was twenty-eight years old and at age twelve had the misfortune of becoming afflicted with serious asthma. For over ten years she lived a difficult life, in constant need of medicine. She had searched all around for a doctor and received all kinds of treatments for asthma, but no positive results were ever obtained. After she got married, her condition unexpectedly became even more serious. At times, she was gasping in a way that was simply unendurable. Cui Ping was completely discouraged about her disease. She didn't want to become a

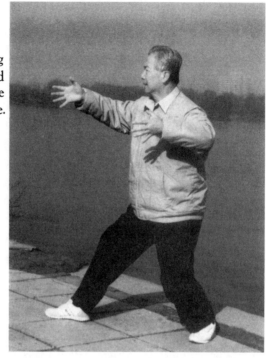

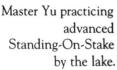

Master Yu practicing advanced Standing-On-Stake by the lake.

burden on her family. One day the thought of throwing her life away came to her. Without the slightest hesitation, she jumped from an upper story of a building.

When she regained consciousness in the hospital, she learned that because she broke a bone in her lumbar vertebra, she was paralysed below the waist. She didn't want to be cured anymore, and she stealthily unscrewed the light switch at the head of the hospital bed, planning to end her life through electrocution. Fortunately, she was discovered by a nurse before a tragedy happened. Under the meticulous healing and care of the army doctors and nurses, Cui Ping's fracture and paralysis were cured, but the terrible asthma demon still kept her tightly in its clutches. She told her husband not to protect her constantly, because she didn't want to live any longer. His wife's words deeply tore the heart of the husband, who loved her very dearly. Was it true that they would let the demon sickness break up this happy family? He heard from a doctor of the miraculous healing of Demon-Palm Huang. Cui Ping and her husband took a train to Shanghai. By the time this couple found Huang Ren-chong, Cui Ping was running out of breath. Huang Ren-chong realized the situation and immediately aimed his chi toward an acupuncture point on Cui's neck. After ten minutes Cui Ping's asthma gradually disappeared. The husband and the wife couldn't stop thanking him. They remained in Shanghai, and after fifteen treatments of external chi, Cui Ping's asthma was cured at its root, and has never recurred to this day.

Is the ability to cure a disease without touching the patient "magic"? "Demon-Palm" refers to the chi gong practitioner's release of energy through the palm (see chapter 9). Without using medicine, without using needles, and without touching the patient, it can cure certain illnesses, even some complicated diseases. This existed among the people in China long ago, in ancient times, but because of its extraordinary nature, and because people didn't understand the logic of its ability to heal, it became shrouded in mysticism, and the people who practiced it were called Demon-Palms.

Since 1974, Huang Ren-chong has used Empty Force chi gong external chi therapy to cure asthma, full and partial paralysis, heart disease, arthritis, sciatic neuralgia, intense headaches, concussions, and other conditions.

Lin Hou-sheng, of Shanghai, presently between age forty-five and fifty, is now teaching chi gong in Hong Kong. I met him in 1984 in Hong Kong, with *Ming Pao Daily* editor Zhang Jing-yun and Suchiro Myles, M.D., and requested that he demonstrate his famous external chi. At that time, standing at a distance of five to six feet from me, he released external chi from two of his fingers toward my back. After about one minute, a small area of my back became warm. This was in the summer, and I was wearing very light clothing. Mr. Zhang and Dr. Myles witnessed that the clothing on the warm area of my back was moving, as if blown by a breeze.

Lin Hou-sheng was the first chi gong master to have his external chi measured with instruments at the Shanghai Atomic Energy Institute. They determined that his chi was infrared. With this test, Chinese scientists verified again and again that chi is a substance. Thus, they realized that it was possible to build a device to imitate the chi of a chi gong master. Because a chi gong master's reserve of chi is limited, releasing too much external chi can be harmful to his health. If it could be reproduced by a machine and produced in high volume, the therapeutic effect of such machines could rival that of actual chi gong masters. At the present time, Chinese scientific research units have built seven different kinds of chi gong devices. Two of these were based on findings derived from measurement of Lin Hou-sheng's chi. For instance, the Sum Li manufacturing company in Guangzhou (Canton) in cooperation with the Guangdong Provincial Qi Gong Scientific Research Organization has produced the Q-2 electronic chi gong master[2] in 1985. This machine was evaluated by the Guandong Provincial Health Department, which issued the following report:

> Electronic chi gong master model Q-2 is based on a study of the working principles of chi gong. The instrument, small in size and simple to operate, has healing and health-preserving capabilities and is deeply appreciated by patients. In tests by the Guangzhou City Main Electronic Industrial Company Product Testing Division, it has completely satisfied the technical specifications of its original design.
>
> In experimental checks on clinical results in the Affiliated Hospital of the Guangzhou College of Traditional Chinese Medicine, the Affiliated Hospital of the Guangdong Province Traditional Chinese Medicine Hospital, the Department of Physical Medicine and Rehabilitation of the First Affiliated Hospital of

Zongshan University of Medicine, the Guangdong Province Pharmacology and Acupuncture Research Center, the Optometry and Opthalmology Department of the Guangzhou Red Cross Hospital, the Acupuncture Department of the Guangzhou City Chinese Medicine Hospital, the Dongshan Region Chinese Medicine and Acupuncture Outpatient Clinic, and the Yuexie Region Bone-Setting Hospital, it was found to have a rate of effectiveness of 86.43% in 505 cases of treatment of arthritis of the shoulder area, work-related injuries of the hip muscles, diseases of the cervical vertebrae, torticollis, sunken occiput, neuralgia of the hipbone, headaches, trigeminal neuralgia, stomach aches, toothaches, tennis elbow, rheumatism, nearsightedness, injury of the cartilage structure, insomnia, and the promotion of health and well-being.

Here follow excerpts from summaries of the clinical results in some of the participating hospitals:

Guangdong Province Pharmacology and Acupuncture Center: [It] is clearly effective in curing nearsightedness, especially pseudo-nearsightedness and nearsightedness under 200 degrees. It produces marked improvement in neuralgia of the eye socket and eyestrain caused by poor vision. *The First Affiliated Hospital of Zonshan Medical College:* . . . our hospital used [it] for healing in twenty cases of work-related injury, convulsions, and injury of the cartilage structure. Of these, three were cured, three showed clear positive effects, ten showed some effects, three showed no effects and one did not complete the treatment. *The Guangdong Province Traditional Chinese Medicine Hospital:* We observed a total of thirty-nine cases with twelve diseases. It was effective in thirty-four cases, and ineffective in five, for an overall rate of effectiveness of 87.2%. Among these, the best effectiveness was found for contusions of the cartilage structure and simple neuralgia. *Donshan Region Chinese Medicine and Acupuncture Outpatient Clinic:* In a study of 121 cases . . . [of] . . . hypertrophy of the cervical and lumbar vertebrae, work-related injury of the hip muscles, sprains, arthritis, headaches and dizziness, heart palpitation, stomach aches, insomnia, coughing . . . [the] overall rate of effectiveness was 95%. *The Acupuncture Department of the Guangzhou City Chinese Medicine Hospital*: Patient Liao, female, seventy-six years old . . . had been feeling intermittent pain in the tips of her toes for more than two years. For the last month the pain was constant, affecting her daily activities and her sleep. A checkup by an outside hospital called it peripheral neuritis, but treatment was ineffective. On January 4, 1985 treatment was applied [by the electronic chi gong master] to the acupuncture points *jiexi* and *taichong* [bilateral]. After two treatments the pain was reduced . . . , after nine treatments, the pain was completely gone. In one month of follow-up, there was no relapse. [3]

Lin Hou-sheng was also the first chi gong master to use external chi as an anesthetic for patients undergoing surgery. We have all heard of acupuncture anesthesia; external chi anesthesia produces its effect with the same technique, aiming external chi toward the relevant acupuncture point and sending it inside the body. Lin Hou-sheng succeeded in giving external chi anesthesia for an excision of a thyroid gland tumor on the morning of May 9, 1980, in the operating room of Shanghai People's Hospital Number Eight. The surgeon in charge of this operation, the chief physician of external medicine, was Mao Huan-yang. During the two-hour operation, the blood pressure was stable and the patient experienced no pain. After that, Lin Hou-sheng performed the same kind of anesthesia in twenty-five cases at Shanghai Sunrise Hospital, Zhuhai City People's Hospital in Guangdong Province, and Shanghai Hospital Number One, and was successful in all cases. Among these were nineteen thyroid gland tumor excisions, three gastrectomies, and three thoracostomies. Lin Hou-sheng's writings include *Qi Gong Makes People Healthy*, published in August 1984 by Guangdong Science and Technology Publishers, and *Qi Gong is the Answer to Health*, of which the first edition of 150,000 copies sold out in one month in 1985.

Wang Rui-ting, formerly living in Shanghai, is now teaching chi gong and healing patients at the Bei Da He Chi Gong Clinic. His Shaolin Internal Energy of One-Finger Art, famous all over China, differs from that of Liu Yong-yen (as discussed in chapter 9). Master Wang does not touch the patient's body while healing, while Master Liu does.

The Internal Energy of One-Finger Art originated in Shaolin Monastery, Fujian Province. Master Wang belongs to the third generation of disciples of this art. His teacher, Master Que Ash-ui (1909–1982) entered Shaolin Monastery at the age of seven and was accepted as a disciple of Du Shun-biao, then master of the monastery, and later became his adopted son. After eighteen years of rigorous training Master Que commanded the Internal Energy of One-Finger Art. He affected many "miraculous" cures throughout his life, saving countless critically ill patients.

Master Wang Rui-ting became a student of Master Que in 1963 and studied with him for ten years. Because of the astonishing effectiveness of his One-Finger Art he became well known and opened a chi gong clinic in Shanghai. His patients have ranged from high officials to ordinary citizens and included people who had been given up repeatedly by Western and traditional Chinese medicine practitioners. This led to requests for him to teach One-Finger Art chi gong, which he now does in Bei Da He as well as all over China.

As a way of illustrating the power of Master Wang I present a 1986 testimony by Guo Qi-di, a surgeon at Qinghai College of Chinese Traditional Medicine.

> I am forty-nine years old, a surgeon who has practiced for over twenty years and cured countless patients. However, when I had an accidental injury myself and suffered traumatic paraplegia as well as serious pain, my colleagues and I were at a loss of what to do. By coincidence, I became acquainted with the uncanny power of One-

Finger Art chi gong and was saved from suffering and a hopeless future. The wonderfully rapid effectiveness of this strange healing technique is amazing.

On June 30, 1986, due to my carelessness while riding a bicycle, I suffered multiple fractures all over the body and became a paraplegic. I was moaning in pain and every day seemed like a year. Even after undergoing forty days of intensive treatments of various types, I still could not sit up. Meanwhile, the Provincial Department of Health invited the chi gong Master Wang Rui-ting from Shanghai to lecture. Thus I was given the opportunity to undergo Master Wang's chi gong healing.

The Master visited me while I was lying flat in bed in the operating room of the Qinghai Province College of Traditional Chinese Medicine. Master Wang started a conversation with me as if I were an old friend he had not seen for a long time. He was full of smiles and kindness and this made me feel a closeness and warmth which could not be compared to anything I had experienced before. While the Master was conversing, he was releasing healing chi at the same time. I had never seen or heard of this healing method before. To all appearances, it was more of a white magic show than a treatment. The Master had been seated by my bed for no more than five minutes, when I began to feel a warm glow and started sweating a little bit. My broken right leg started to have slight tinges of burning, numbness, and swelling, and it felt as if ants were crawling over my skin. At the same time I felt a cold air rising from the sole of the feet, as if pulled by some invisible force. Gradually I began to feel tiny needles sticking in my feet in an unbearably painful way. Then I suddenly heard the stunned exclamations of the medical staff observing the scene: "The leg is rising!" I turned to look at them. They were all transfixed, and I also was stunned to see that it was true, my paralyzed foot was miraculously rising. It was a mixture of astonishment and thrill for me. I noticed Master Wang raising his hand, and just like a marionette pulled by invisible strings, my leg moved whichever way the Master moved his hand. When the Master's hand went to the right, my leg went to the right; when the hand moved left, my leg followed left! My leg was under his control, under his command. "Wang is a Master of Black Magic," I thought, but then, "No!" All this was too unthinkable, too mysterious.

Master Wang treated me five times. Now, not only can I walk, I can also go out for a stroll and even climb four flights of stairs. I could not have imagined this when not long ago I was moaning with pain in bed. There were no words to express my gratitude to the Master. I will never forget the happiness and health the Master brought me. As a surgeon specializing in traumatology, whose family has a tradition of practicing traumatology, I can only feel very stirred by this dreamlike experience I went through.[4]

Liu Han-wen is sixty-five years old and retired. Born in Shandong Province, he was involved in professional health care activities for thirty years. He was vice-chairman and general secretary of the Liaoning Province Working Committee for the Popularization of Qi Gong. In 1958, he was selected as a committee member of the Committee for the National Martial Arts Association. All his life he has practiced the Secret Law Chi Gong which was passed down to him from his ancestors. He has practiced for fifty years and his force is remarkable. In August 1983, the Metal Research Institute of the Chinese Academy of Sciences selected two males and two females who had never had any contact with chi gong, and Master Liu was able to cause in them marked changes in selected physiological and biophysical indicators whenever he wanted, sending external chi from a distance of fifteen and thirty meters through a partition forty centimeters thick. Over a period of thirty years, he has cured tens of thousands of patients with external chi. The person he cures need not be in the same place with him. He can transmit "information" to cure a disease from miles away. The patient specifies the time and direction beforehand, and the patient can receive the information transfer and be cured whenever he wishes. Liu Han-wen's chi gong power transforms from the chi gong quiet state into a psychic state.

He often gives public demonstrations of a mass of chi released from the top of his head. At least two-thirds of the audience sees a misty gas rising from his head. It never ceases to amaze people. In addition, several times he has done a test in which he sends external chi at students living in different parts of the same city. All of them received his information transfer; some smelled a characteristic scent, some were completely immersed in chi, some began swinging around uncontrollably, and some wouldn't stop smiling until he stopped releasing external chi.

Among the most objective and incontrovertible research findings reported are those of three researchers from the Metallurgy Research Institute of the Chinese Academy of Sciences, Huang Li, Lin Xue-rong, and Xu Jun. On March 20, 1982, at the invitation of the Shenyang City Qi Gong Research Institute, they conducted experiments on chi gong masters releasing energy and the excitation of the recipients of the energy with the AGA Thermovision 780 infrared heat imaging system.

When Master Liu released his energy, the spread of high temperature states in his palms was observed. During the second to the fifth minutes of his release, the infrared radiation of his palm and forearm increased and when the number of high-temperature points gradually increased, they joined in lines and the high temperature spread to all five fingers. At this time the highest temperature increase measured in the area was .5°.[5] When Master Liu interrupted his energy release, the high-temperature spots on the fingertips and palms gradually disappeared.

When a chi gong master releases healing energy to a patient, the recipient of the energy often reports feelings of warmth, swelling, itching, and tingling. These feelings are associated with the chi transmission process. In order to verify this with Master Liu, the researchers selected a person unfamiliar with chi gong and had him stand at a distance of twenty meters. Before Master Liu released his energy, the temperature of his hands, fingers, and forearms were measured and they showed no change over a period of five minutes. Three minutes after Master Liu had started releasing energy the temperature of his palms and the surrounding areas had increased, and the temperature at the point of greatest heat was raised .4°. The main feeling reported by the recipient of the energy, twenty meters removed, was one of warmth.

Another report on the abilities of Master Liu was provided in *Kaifeng Technology* of June 25, 1986:

> On May 28, the Kaifeng City District Army Auditorium was jampacked. On the podium stood Liu Han-wen, practitioner of chan mystery [secret law] chi gong. He held a 2.5-inch-long silver needle between thumb and forefinger, which he pointed at the right *hegu* acupuncture point of Dai Feng-ying, over fifty years old. A short time afterward, the needle started twirling and moving up and down, as if it were a real operation. The point of the silver needle always remained five or six inches above the skin, but the target [the skin *hegu* point] was visibly moving up and down. The performer of the operation moved the needle along the meridians and finally up to the *bai-hui* acupoint on the crown of the head. The right part of Dai's body followed the constantly glittering motions of the needle. After Master Liu put away the needle, tears welled up in the patient's eyes. The right half of his body, which had been deadened to all sensations for five years, felt warm, and he could use his hemiparetic right leg and right arm much better than before.
>
> Afterward, Comrade Yu Zhao-mei, vice-chairman of the City Science Association, stood up in the crowd. He described a spot on the outside of his left leg, the size of a fist, which had been devoid of all sensations for three years and which acupuncture and electric therapy had failed to cure. After hearing this, Master Liu nodded his assent for the man to climb up on the square bench, let his feet and legs dangle naturally, and close his eyes. Then Master Liu began moving his palms to the diseased spot for short periods. After two minutes, the audience saw the muscles of the patient twitching. Liu Han-wen asked the patient what he felt. Yu Zhao-mei

pinched the deadened spot and said happily: "It worked; I can feel pain in this part of the body now!"

Yan Xin of Chongqing City, Sichuan Province is thirty-six years old. He graduated from Chengdu College of Traditional Chinese Medicine, and at present he serves in the Chongqing Institute of Traditional Chinese Medicine. In his childhood he studied martial arts and chi gong under the famous master of martial arts Hai Deng. After practicing diligently for ten years, he derived psychic powers from chi gong. He often performs healings, and his patients recover every time. He is famous all over the country and is called a "miracle doctor." In recognition of his gifts, the Chinese government has designated him a "National Treasure." The noted Beijing newspaper *Guangming Daily* also praised him as "packing together Chinese traditional medicine, qi gong, martial arts and psychic powers in one body." In the period from 1987 to 1988, over four hundred different newspapers and magazines have reported about him. Thousands have heard his lectures. Wherever he goes and gives a lecture, he usually draws an audience of between five thousand and seven thousand people; the most he ever drew was thirty thousand people. Why do so many people come to hear his lectures? It is said that when patients listen to his lecture, their diseases go away automatically. A healthy person who listens to his lecture will have increased energy. A considerable number of people experience spontaneous shaking and start moving around. Mainland China has a term, "external chi induced movement," which means that people, who feel the chi which is sent, will be caused to move. For this reason, researchers from the High Energy Physics Research Institute of the Chinese Academy of Science, set up instruments to register the chi field when Master Liu was lecturing. The instruments registered light and high energy neutrons as well as a strong magnetic field on the sites where he was lecturing.[6]

Today, China has about three thousand chi gong masters. Of the seven masters described above, I am personally acquainted with all except Wang Rui-tin and Yan Xin, and I regularly have contact with all of them by mail. They are the most famous chi gong masters in mainland China today. However, China is a vast land with a huge population, and among its one billion people, perhaps there exists someone with even higher powers than Yan Xin.

Notes

1. A nonmalignant breast tumor of fibrous and glandular tissue. Because the tumor may grow to a large size and could then be disfiguring, and also may become cancerous, many doctors advise surgical removal.

2. According to Mr. Young Xiao-bin, director of the Guangdong Qi Gong Scientific Research Center, more than one million of these machines were sold. The machine is available in the U.S., and Paul Dong owns one for research purposes.

3. Guandong Provincial Health Department, Guangzhou: Untitled Report 7/25/85.

4. Guo Qi-di, in Wang Rui-ting: *One-Finger Art of Shaolin Temple* (Xian: Shansi Science and Technology Publ.) Oct. 1987, p. 91.

5. Paul Dong repeated the same thermography tests on himself in San Francisco in 1989 after receiving a copy of Master Liu's book, *Secret Law of Chi Gong*. Dong followed the instructions and performed the suggested chi gong exercises. A copy of his test results, measured by Computerized Thermographic Imaging, Inc., on May 18, 1989, is available on request.

6. See for example, Wang Yao-lan, Lu Zu-yin, and Yan Xin in "A Method of Detecting Qi Field" (Abstract describing measurements made on October 8, 1987, in the auditorium of the Institute of Political Sciences, Beijing, and on October 21, 1987, in the Hongqijie Auditorium).

8

How to Perform Chi Gong

Great accomplishments are possible
With attention to small beginnings.

—Lao Tzu, *Tao Te Ching*, 63

About twenty million people in China practice chi gong. More than one hundred types of chi gong are common, falling into three broad categories: still exercises, moving exercises, and a combination of these two, still-and-moving exercises. Although the different schools of chi gong training have their respective idiosyncrasies, all methods involve breath, thought, and body parts.

The training of spirit and thought is to "quiet the mind," or enter into a state of meditation. In this state one practices *the control of thought,* which requires concentration in order for the cerebral cortex to be in a highly focused state. It is also called the internal guarding of thought.

The training of breathing, that is, *the control of breath,* consists of the following principal methods: exhaling, inhaling, and the various ways of blowing—*xu* (breathing out or hissing slowly), *chui* (blowing out or puffing), *he* (breathing out with the mouth open), and *si* (hissing).

The training of body parts, that is, *the control of postures,* consists of six principal forms: walking, standing, sitting, lying, kneeling, and massaging.

125

Regardless of the chi gong training method adopted, the trainee will succeed in attaining chi gong skills if he or she sticks to it under strict guidance.

Chi gong exercises of the *still* type generally are best for elderly people; *moving* exercises are better suited for the young; those of the combined still-and-moving type are best for the middle-aged. However, there is no hard and fast rule about this. Some older people find it difficult to go into the state of stillness; they therefore should practice moving exercises. Likewise, some young people, if quiet by nature, may be inclined to practice still exercises. Experience indicates that one kind of chi gong may not suit every person. In this case, a switch to another kind is recommended, until a suitable kind of exercise is found. The key for choosing the right form of chi gong is to determine whether it induces a true sense of comfort and well-being. If the trainee cannot understand the procedure of the exercise, he or she will be distracted by thinking about what to do next. In such a case the mind will not go easily into the exercise, and we advise the trainee to choose a simpler kind of chi gong.

We will present two simple, but extremely powerful, still exercises—Standing-on-Stake chi gong and Relaxed and Quiet chi gong—suitable for just about everyone except pregnant women. Chi gong practice should preferably be performed while standing in the north-south orientation, because of the Chinese belief in keeping oneself aligned with the earth's magnetic field.

Standing-On-Stake Chi Gong

Inspired by the natural phenomenon of a stationary tree continually growing and developing, the Taoist philosopher Wang Chongyang invented the Standing-On-Stake exercise approximately two thousand years ago. Its therapeutic effect results from the fact that it keeps the limbs bent at a certain angle so that the tendons and muscles are kept in a state of continuous contraction, thereby promoting the redistribution of blood throughout the body. Blood circulation is stimulated, especially within the internal organs, and the blood capillaries are opened to a larger extent. According to Master Yu Yong-nian (introduced in chapter 7), performing the Standing-On-Stake exercise for an hour—the amount he exercises each time—can increase red blood cells by 1.5 million, white blood cells by 3,600, and hemoglobin by 3.2 grams in every cubic centimeter of blood. Hemoglobin, of course, is the oxygen carrier within the body, bringing it to tissues and organs, thereby causing improvement in the functioning of the entire body. Try a simple test:

Stand for twenty minutes with your arms and legs unbent, then for twenty minutes with arms and legs bent. In the latter case, your hands and legs will warm up because the bending causes your blood to circulate faster. According to traditional Chinese medicine, non-circulation causes pain. When circulation of the blood is blocked to some degree, not only is pain caused, but diseases also occur.[1]

The following are simple if subtle chi gong exercises that can be practiced anywhere at any time. Ideally, these should be performed three times a day for twenty minutes each. However, beginners may not have enough strength in the legs, so one might want to start with five minute sessions. Add five minutes each week until the twenty minute level is reached.

Posture One (fig. 8-1)

In this exercise it is sufficient to keep breathing naturally, as one would during the activities of everyday life. This means that the trainee should *not* think about breathing in any special way, for instance, breathing deeply, or visualizing the chi collecting at the *dan tian* point, as recommended in advanced chi gong exercises.

1. Stand upright in a natural posture, quiet and relaxed with your legs apart at shoulder width.
2. Bend both legs slightly, so that your knees do not extend beyond the tips of your toes.
3. Raise both hands lightly, with fingers spread and palms down, until your forearms are parallel to the ground.
4. Close your eyes and concentrate on the area just below your navel, the *dan tian*. In the beginning stages you might touch the *dan tian* as many times as needed to remind yourself where the area is, but then you should be able to, as the masters say, "listen to, think about, and pay attention to" the *dan tian*. Hold this position until the end of the exercise. (If you find it difficult to focus your mind on the navel, you may open your eyes to gaze on a distant object or view. When practicing indoors you may fix your attention on an object or spot on the opposite wall without concentrating on the navel.)

Ending the Standing-On-Stake Exercise

1. To end the exercise, slowly open your eyes and let your body resume a fully upright posture.

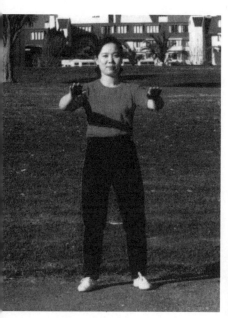

Standing-On-Stake, posture 1.
Front and side view.

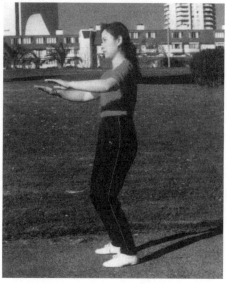

2. Rub your hands to warm them and then use them to wipe your face twelve times.[2] Place the palms over your eyes and then lightly wipe the palms from the front of your face to the back of your neck.

3. Take a stroll for ten minutes or so.

Posture Two (fig. 8-2)

This is the same as posture one except that you place your hands about one foot in front with the palms facing the navel and the fingertips of each hand pointing at those of the other as in the figure.

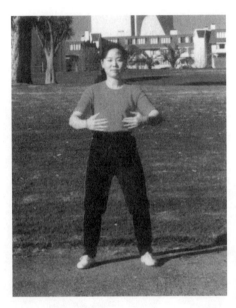

Standing-On-Stake, posture 2.
Front and side view.

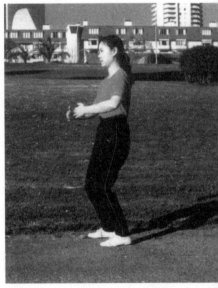

Posture Three (fig. 8-3)

This is the same as posture one except that you place your hands about one foot in front with the palms facing the chest and the fingertips of one hand pointing at those of the other as in the figure.

Practice posture one for three months, go on to posture two for three months, and, after that, posture three for another three months. After nine months of practice, combine all three postures into one daily half-hour session in which you practice each posture for ten minutes, starting with posture one.

Do not be misled by the apparent plainness of Standing-On-Stake. Though it appears so, it is by no means easy. Paul Dong's teacher, Master Yu Yong-nian, in his book *A Way To Prolong Life* describes Standing-On-Stake as "a motion exercise that has no motion." He says, "Although the tree is stationary, yet it continues to live, ever growing and developing, toughening and expanding."

Relaxed and Quiet Chi Gong

Set the time for this exercise at half an hour. You can perform this exercise from either a standing or sitting position (using the front third of the chair). If you have no difficulties, standing throughout is recommended.

1. Stand still and relaxed with your arms hanging down. Clear all distracting thoughts from your mind. Relax all over, then shut your eyes and lower your head (to align your *bai-hui* point, see next chapter).
2. Fix your attention on the navel by using your left hand to touch your navel three times. Then stand quietly for a little while.

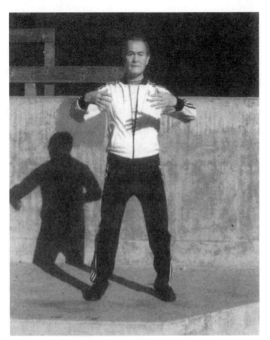

Standing-On-Stake, posture 3.

Front and side view of group exercise.

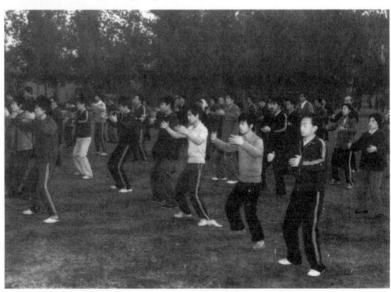

3. Take a dozen deep breaths, inhaling and exhaling deeply twelve times.

4. Imagine that you are looking at your eyes and then at the *zuqiao* acupoint located between the eyes (see fig. 8-4) for one second. Imagine the chi traveling from the acupoint all the way down to the navel. When it reaches the navel hold the image for three breaths (a complete inhalation and exhalation make one breath).

5. Visualize yourself breathing through your navel for five times. For each breath, visualize your navel and the *ming men* acupoint (on your back opposite the navel) sticking together.

6. Visualize yourself inhaling through the *ming men* acupoint for five times, exactly as you did for the navel in step 5.

7. For the next ten to fifteen minutes, gently and effortlessly fix your thoughts on your navel and listen to your inhalation and exhalation. When listening to your breath do not intentionally make it sound louder or influence it in any way.

Ending the Relaxed and Quiet Exercise

This five minute portion must be done standing.

1. First suggest to yourself that you are going to end the exercise. Then slowly open your eyes and lift your head to the upright position. Gaze at a distant object or view for a while.

2. Use your left hand to stroke your abdomen around the navel twenty-four times in ever increasing circles. Let your thoughts follow your action.

3. Repeat step 2 but stroke in the opposite direction.

4. Rub both hands together in front of your chest until they become warm. Then use them to wipe your face thirty-six times in the manner described in Standing-On-Stake.

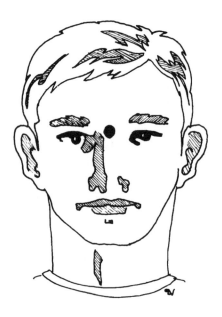

The *zuqiao* acupoint.

5. Use your right hand to pat your left shoulder three times. Then use your left hand for patting your right shoulder in like manner.
6. Use your right hand to tap your left hand from top to bottom three times, then do the same with your left hand to pat the right.
7. Bending over, pat your feet three times from top to bottom; use your right hand for the left and your left hand for the right foot. Then straighten up.

The Relaxed and Quiet Exercise should be practiced twice a day, each time for half an hour, or once a day for an hour.

Spontaneous Movement

Whether you take the standing or sitting posture, *stillness in the extreme will lead to motion.* It seems odd, but profound mental and physical quiet, with the body relaxed throughout, will make your blood and chi flow more quickly. The process will eventually lead to a spontaneous natural swinging motion of the body. Generally, it takes at least three months of training before sufficient stillness is reached for the swinging motion to emerge in a practice session. For every ten people who practice, five will probably be able to achieve the swinging motion. When it occurs, do not try to control it. Just let yourself swing freely until you choose to end the exercise. At that point you should firmly will the motion to stop *before* ending the exercise.

It is thought that spontaneous movement is related to bursts of chi energy circulating through the body and that for it to occur at least the small circuit (see chapter 3) would have been activated. The occurrence of spontaneous movement is therefore considered to be a sign of progress, and the student could at this time attempt to master the activation of the small circuit. Paul Dong has been practising chi gong for ten years and his experience confirms the ancient observations of the circulation of chi energy. According to Dong:

> The kind of chi gong I practice is called the spontaneous movement. After only three months training, I found that whenever I stood still and relaxed I entered into a state of deep tranquility. When I guard my *dan tian* point for fifteen minutes, the body begins to move automatically. That is, the internal chi (or energy within) is aroused and flows through my entire body, causing the body and limbs to move spontaneously. As is claimed by chi gong practitioners, I have found that when chi is flowing within the body it will cause a feeling of swelling, numbness, soreness, or ache, or the phenomenon of patting.[3] When chi comes across a weak or

unbalanced place (a center of illness), an automatic massage of the internal organs will occur and the illness will be ameliorated or cured.

Although we know that automatic movement or patting may also be caused by self-suggestion or self-hypnosis, the reader should realize that these subjective phenomena are part and parcel of a total change which Dong has experienced after he began the practice of chi gong. These feelings are real and reveal a positive benefit of chi gong caused by a change in the mind-set of the practitioners. Even if the effects Dong describes can be successfully accomplished by self-hypnosis of millions of chi gong practitioners from all walks of life, it should appeal to Americans. After all, millions in our country have benefited from less ancient and experimentally researched self-suggestion practices as evidenced by the success of such books as Norman Vincent Peale's *The Power of Positive Thinking*.

Establishing the Practice Routine

Choose either one of the above stationary exercises (or any of those discussed in other chapters) and practice it diligently. Usually the effect will become obvious only after one hundred days of uninterrupted practicing.

Before beginning a practice session you should prepare yourself in various ways. Go to the bathroom first, so your bowel and bladder will not require your attention. Wear shoes, socks, and loose garments during practice; do not constrict your body with tight clothing, but keep warm at all times when practicing chi gong. If you feel hungry before a session, take a light meal, or a glass of warm water, milk, or clear soup. You should not have sexual relations for an hour before and afterward. Also, do not drink alcoholic beverages for an hour before. Make certain you will not be disturbed by telephones ringing. Turn off any electrical appliances that might disturb you.

Chi gong is suitable for men and women, young and old, but there are certain exceptions: severely disturbed mental patients, pregnant women, and people suffering from acute infectious diseases. In cases of internal bleeding, nosebleeds, or bleeding after tooth extractions or trauma, you should avoid exercising. Also abstain from exercising if you menstruate, feel dizzy, or have a fever. The reasons are simply that chi gong makes the blood and chi circulate more vigorously, and thus bleeding due to trauma or menstruation may be unduly prolonged. Feeling dizzy is a contraindication to any exercise, and chi gong is no exception. Also, if you are physically ill or feverous you will not benefit from chi gong.

According to ancient tradition, the best time for chi gong exercises are 3 to 5 A.M., 11 A.M. to 1 P.M., and 11 P.M. to 1 A.M. If none of these hours suit you, choose any hour that does and then adhere to it as a fixed hour, dedicated to your practice. In other words, be regular about your sessions. Form a habit and hold to it. In the summer, it is nice to perform chi gong outdoors along a river or a lake, in the forest or mountains, or in the shadow of a tree. Ancient tradition holds that the shadow of a pine tree is particularly conducive to effective practice—perhaps because pine trees give off large amounts of oxygen. Another ancient secret of chi gong is that exercise is particularly effective for three days before and after the full moon. Modern physiological research indicates that the moon's gravitational effect quickens or retards blood circulation. Perhaps that is the reason behind this bit of ancient lore.

When someone is resolved to succeed in mastering chi gong or when a patient is strongly motivated to restore his or her health as soon as possible, it is best to practice in the open country rather than a built-up area. In a city, air pollution and magnetic fields from electrical wires and appliances are everywhere; these are bound to be somewhat deleterious to health. A popular story provides an instructive example of this principle: Legend has it that a monk brought up in the mountains became a master of chi gong. One day he went to Shanghai, one of the world's largest cities. Upon arrival he felt quite weak and lost some of his power and skill in chi gong. But once he left the city and returned to the mountains, he immediately regained all of his mastery.

This story may be fanciful exaggeration, but it dramatizes the point about your personal power and the effect of negative influences on your chi gong practice. Seek the countryside whenever possible, just as astronomers build their observatories away from cities to avoid the interference of light on their instruments. For people practicing chi gong, the instrument is their body. The principle is the same: Avoid or minimize whatever unhealthy interference there may be around you.[4]

How to Develop External Chi

Paul Dong believes that the capability to release external chi is only possible after the student has mastered the activation of the small circuit (see chapter 3). The student can then proceed to activate the large circuit by adding the following exercises (Steps Toward Release of External Chi) to the daily practice of Standing-On-Stake chi gong.

1. Follow the Standing-on Stake postures provided earlier and practice these for twelve minutes.
2. External Chi Step 1: Now assume posture one except that you place your hands with their palms facing one another approximately two feet in front of your chest (fig. 8-5).
3. External Chi Step 2: Same as step 1, but place your left hand about four inches from your navel with the palm up, and your

right hand about four inches from your chest with the palm down (fig. 8-6).

4. External Chi Step 3: Repeat as before in step 2, but reverse the position of the hands.

5. External Chi Step 4: Place your left leg about one and a half feet in front of your right leg. Bend your left leg until the knee is even with the tips of the toes. Raise your left hand above the shoulder so that the palm faces the sky. Hold the right hand beside the right leg with the palm facing the ground (fig. 8-7).

6. External Chi Step 5: Repeat as before in step 4, but reverse the position of the legs and hands (fig. 8-8).

End the exercise in the same manner as the Standing-On-Stake exercise.

Practice these additional five external chi steps for at least one hour daily, beginning with practicing each of the steps for two minutes and adding one minute each week, until you spend twelve minutes on each of the steps. Focus half of the time on your navel and the other half of the time on your palms. If you want to use your index (or index and middle) finger(s) in guiding external chi (see chapter 9), concentrate one-third of your practice time on your navel, your palms, and your fingers respectively.

When you become powerful enough to guide your external chi (after at least one year's daily practice), activate your large circuit (see fig. 3-2, p. 71) by imagining it as going straight down from the *dan tian* to the *yong quan* point (located at the sole of your feet) and up the back of the body. From there it goes up to the *da zhui* point (located low in the neck between your shoulders) and then down to both your palms and your fingers before it returns to your *dan tian*.

We advise against practicing release of external chi unless under the direction of a chi gong master associated with a licensed medical doctor, to oversee any intended healing.[5]

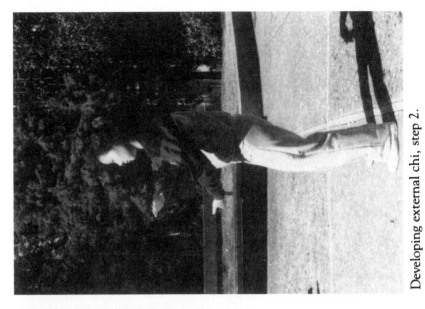

Developing external chi, step 2.

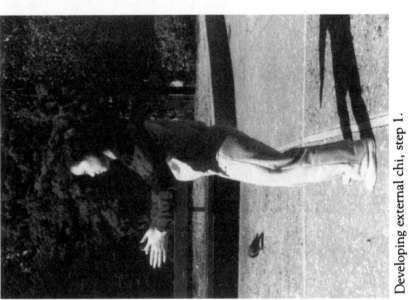

Developing external chi, step 1.

140

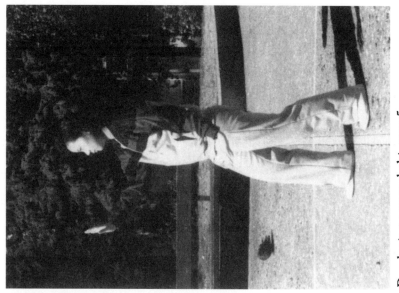

Developing external chi, step 5.

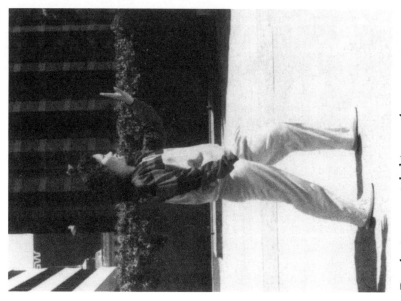

Developing external chi, step 4.

141

Notes

1. Paul Dong has practiced the Standing-On-Stake exercise for more than five years and has succeeded in curing or greatly alleviating every one of the diseases afflicting him prior to the practice of chi gong (see chapter 4). He feels that Standing-On-Stake chi gong is so beneficial that he now teaches a class on it at the YMCA in San Francisco.

2. The number of times recommended for repeating different aspects of the chi gong practice sequence is determined by each master's style. In this book we follow the original instructions Paul Dong was given by the masters who taught him.

3. The phenomenon of spontaneously patting yourself, for instance, on the thigh.

4. Chi is related to electromagnetic energy fields. In the last decade, the potential health hazards of electric power sources has been recognized, and it is clear that electrical fields around power lines, household wiring, and electric appliances can interfere with the activation of chi. Exactly this possibility was addressed in a recent article by scientists from the Massachusetts Institute of Technology and the National Institute of Standards and Technology. They concluded that "concerns related to possible biological effects due to very weak environmental electrical fields cannot be dismissed on the grounds of being swamped by thermal fluctuations." J. C. Weaver and R. D. Astumian, "The Response of Living Cells to Very Weak Electric Fields," *Science* 247 (1990): 459–61.

5. The occurrence of quick learning of external chi release, even in young children after a few days practice, is described in Y. Omura et al., "Unique Changes on the Qi Gong Master's and Patient's Body During Qi Gong Treatment: Their Relationships to Certain Meridians and Acupuncture Points and the Recreation of Therapeutic Qi Gong States by Children and Adults," *Acupuncture and Electro-Therapeutics Research, International Journal* 14 (1989): 61–89. As mentioned in chapters 7 and 9, we think that the practice of chi gong takes time and that it is rarely developed in children. This does not mean that children cannot have strong chi; after all, the recent renaissance of chi began with the discovery of psychic powers in children (see chapter 10). But we do not feel that children can readily develop mastery of the circulation of chi in the small and large circuits as this is required for *consistent* delivery of external chi.

9

The Magic Palm and One-Finger Art

Enough, if something from our hands have power
to live, and act, and serve

—William Wordsworth

In most houses and buildings today, we get water by turning on a faucet and drain it by removing a sink plug. We can use this plumbing analogy to describe the human body, which has many passages everywhere; the nervous system, the circulatory system, and what is known in traditional Chinese medicine as channels or meridians. These systems do not to carry water, but energy (which, as we know from chapter 1 includes substance and information). These systems also have certain points, like faucets, where one can regulate the energy entering or leaving the body.

Traditional Chinese medicine and chi gong specialists hold that energy within the body comes partially from heaven and partially from earth, and is absorbed through the skin, capillaries of the lung and digestive systems, and acupuncture points. Some of the acupoints are particularly sensitive and absorb most of the energy from heaven and earth. These are the *bai-hui*, *yong quan*, *ming men*, and *dan tian* points (see fig. 3-1 and 3-2, pp. 70 and 71). In particular the

143

bai-hui point, like an antenna on the top of the head, plays a vital role. If it is difficult for us to understand how energy is absorbed from heaven and earth, we might think of installations which absorb solar energy.

When a chi gong practitioner stands or sits in order to exercise, he or she is required to have the *bai-hui* point face heaven in order to absorb the greatest possible energy from the universe (*yang* energy). Since the *bai-hui* point is on the crown of the head, it always faces the sky if one is standing or sitting straight, but that does not mean it is at the exact position. The chi gong practitioner must lower his/her head slightly, because the *Bai-hui* point is an inch behind the vertex. When the point aligns perfectly with the sky, it is said that it is wide open to absorb energy from the universe.

Just as the human body can absorb energy, it can also issue and diffuse energy through the skin, capillaries, and acupoints. Some acupoints are particularly capable of issuing energy: the eyes, the fingertips, and the *Laogong* point in the middle of the palm. Therefore, when a chi gong master applies external chi it is always through the eyes, fingertips, or *Laogong* points. The eyes, and in particular the index and middle finger, as well as the *Laogong* point, can be used separately, but generally the eyes in coordination with the finger-points, or the *Laogong* point, are used.

The eyes command the thought while the external energy emanates from the fingers or the *Laogong* point. Whether you are using fingers or the *Laogong* acupoint to issue external chi, the energy called upon is not immediately available. This takes some advanced exercise. Some people practice with their index fingers to issue external chi, and this is called One-Finger Art. Others specialize with the *Laogong* acupoint, and that is called Magic Palm. Internal chi from the chi gong practitioner is released from the finger or the *Laogong* point into an acupuncture point of the subject (a healer knows which acupoint of the patient to use for a specific disease), so

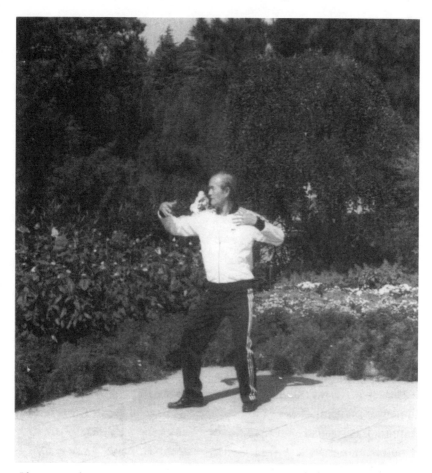

Chi gong close to pine trees for optimal absorption of oxygen. Note the head position with the *bai-hui* acupoint wide open to absorb chi energy.

as to influence the patient's chi. These are the healing skills and powers passed down to chi gong practitioners by their ancestors.

Before training in One-Finger Art or Magic Palm, one needs at least a year's practice in chi gong. In particular, one must have a feeling that the *Dan Tian* region is full of chi and the body filled with energy before chi can be induced and released. Otherwise there will be insufficient energy in the body to release. Those powerful chi gong masters who can heal have practiced for at least three years, some for between ten and twenty years. The longer one practices, the more one is able to invoke and release chi and the stronger the effect.

The Standing-On-Stake method discussed in chapter 8 may be followed for energy release until a strong feeling of energy is produced at the *Laogong* acupoint (as evidenced by the palms feeling hot and numb, and a feeling of attraction between the palms when one puts the hands together). It will take a year or longer before the index finger is capable of releasing chi.

Master Huang Ren-chong, mentioned in chapter 7, specializes in applying external energy through the *Laogong* acupoint of his palm. His superb skill and outstanding healing effects have earned him the venerable title "Demon-Palm Huang." Master Hai Deng of the Shaolin Monastery can stand on one finger[1], which is a form of One-Finger Art. In Xiamen City, Fukien Province, Superintendent Liu Yong-yen of the Chunghua Hospital is also called a chi master of the One-Finger Art, because with his skills, based upon thirty years of experience, he is capable of releasing external chi with his index finger or treating patients by massaging their acupoints, both with remarkable success. Another celebrated chi gong master, Wang Rui-ting of Shanghai, also discussed in chapter 7, is well-known for his One-Finger Art. He teaches his knowledge of the "Shaolin Internal Energy of One Finger Art" at the Bei Da He chi gong clinic, and the China Qi Gong Research Organization often shows him practicing chi gong on the cover of its publications.

Every year over three thousand patients get cured thanks to the One-Finger Art of Liu Yong-yen and Wang Rui-ting, and it is estimated that over one million people are helped yearly by other masters using Magic Palm or One-Finger Art. This is why people say: "Is not the arrangement of God to let our own energy make amends when conventional medicine fails?"

In every skill to be trained, there is a particular aspect to which special attention must be paid. To release energy through the *Laogong* point requires special training of the palm. Likewise, training in One-Finger Art requires special attention to the index finger, as follows:

One-Finger Art (Including a Brief Discussion of Magic Palm)

The student should only start these exercises after he/she has managed to activate the small circuit (chapter 3, figure 3-1) and preferably be guided by a chi gong master in this endeavor.

1. First practice Relaxed and Quiet chi gong for half an hour.
2. Go on to practice Standing-On-Stake for half hour.
3. After the above practice, start touching the palate with the tongue. Raise both hands slowly, empty fists (that is middle finger bent to touch thumb and the index finger pointing up, see finger 9-2) with middle, ring, and little fingers stretching out toward the stomach and both arms bent as high up as the eyes. The index finger should be a foot away from the eyes and at a distance as much as between the pupils of the eyes, from each other. The joints of both elbows should slightly touch the sides of the body and thoughts should be in a state of concentration, i.e., do not let your thoughts wander. Both eyes should stare at the fingertips (see figure 9-3). The duration of sustained concentration may vary individually, but may increase from one to ten minutes.

At first one may have difficulty getting accustomed to holding the above complex posture, but after doing it for some time, one will get used to it. A problem may arise when double images appear; one sees the index fingers turn to four and sometimes eight. Don't panic, persist in training and the

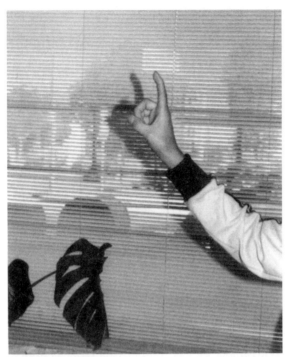

Empty Fist
(also see fig. 9–3).

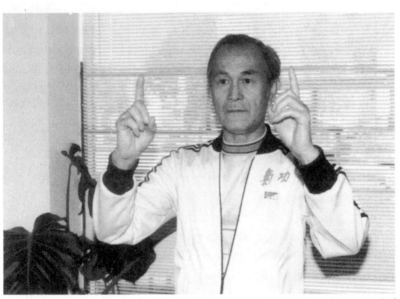

One-Finger Art. Note the upward direction of the index finger and the downward direction (toward the belly) of the other fingers.

double images will automatically disappear. A white substance, resembling smoke may be detected at the finger tips.
When the smoke disappears, there is an indication of white
light at the finger tips.

4. End of exercise: Close the eyes for a while, then open them.
   Rub your hands to make them warm and then use them to
   wipe your face twelve times. Place the palms over your eyes
   and then lightly wipe the palms from the front of your face to
   the back of your neck.

5. Take a stroll for ten minutes or so.

Practice chi gong with patience:

At this point we must emphasize the need to wait for at least one year
before starting the next level of exercise, except in those cases where
the student has been able to master the large circuit quickly. Chi gong
remains a discipline which must be practiced with patience and determination, and one should build its accomplishments step-by-step. If
you start skipping steps while climbing an unfamiliar staircase, you
are likely to stumble or fall. Likewise, if you don't observe the required
stages in the advanced practice of chi gong, not only is there a chance
that you will not benefit at all, but you may even hurt yourself.

After practicing the above exercises until getting results—this
often takes more than one year—add the following exercises after
step 3.

3a. Sit down (posture as in Relaxed and Quiet chi gong), place
    both hands on your loins with Empty Fists (see fig. 9.2, but
    in this case stretching the index fingers toward the belly),
    the fingers being a foot apart and the joints of the elbows
    touching slightly the sides of the body. With eyes closed,
    begin inducing the large circuit circulation of the chi energy
    (fig. 3-2, p. 71).

3b. Experience the energy flowing down the pubic region through the *huiyin* (perineum) acupoint, *yong quan* (sole of the foot) acupoint, and up to the *dazhui* acupoint (at the back of the neck), whence the energy begins to travel in two routes: simultaneously from the *dazhui* point down to the *laogong* point (along both arms) and also to the tips of the index fingers. The exercise takes ten minutes each time, after which you should concentrate your thoughts on the index fingers for another five minutes.

Practice the above exercises for a year and a half to two years, and the One-Finger Art will be achieved. If a strong skill is desired practice for another year with 3a and 3b periods extended after the second year. Of course, exceptional students or those assisted by a chi gong master daily may experience faster results.

There are other kinds of One-Finger Art. In chapter 7 we mentioned the "Shaolin Internal Energy of One Finger Art." Master Wang Rui-ting combines finger-bending exercises with Standing-On-Stake chi gong. The student should practice Standing-On-Stake chi gong for a minimum of six months before beginning the finger-bending exercises. Thereafter one can start with bending the fingers, ten minutes after having begun chi gong and while maintaining the Standing-On-Stake exercise. The finger exercises consist of bending all fingers separately one-by-one starting with the thumbs, as much as possible, with the palms held down. The bending of each finger should total about two minutes and proceed gradually; the finger should be held at its lowest point for a while and then slowly brought back (see fig. 9-4). The recommended frequency of finger bending is: thumbs, once; index fingers, seven times; middle fingers, three times; ring fingers, nine times; and the little fingers, five times.

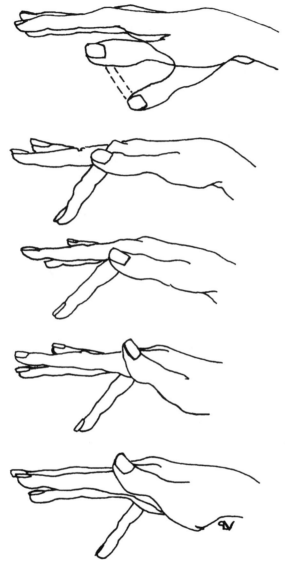

Exercise for Shaolin Internal Energy of One-Finger Art.

Magic Palm

In the chapter 8, when discussing the chi gong to develop external chi we described the additional five steps needed to release chi from the palm of your hand. By concentrating on your *laogong* point for five minutes after each activation of the large circuit you may in time develop the accumulation of chi needed for the power of the Magic Palm.

End all exercises following steps 4 and 5 of the One-Finger Art exercise (p. 149).

What Are the Possible Applications?

The One-Finger Art and Magic Palm are used in therapy, and when successfully trained the fingers can take the place of acupuncture needles with better effect and no pain. As was explained in chapter 3, the underlying principle in all chi gong exercises is the same as in acupuncture. In One-Finger Art the finger may touch or remain half an inch away from the acupoint. But with the Magic Palm the external energy can only be issued when the healer is not touching the acupoint.

External chi from the palm or the fingers may be used for simple self-healing. To begin with, the student should seek advice from a doctor of TCM. Afterward he or she may treat such minor ailments as headaches, colds, arthritis, insomnia, and other minor afflictions by pointing the palm or the fingers at the site, or, if the student has been acquainted with the meridians of Chinese medicine, he or she may apply external chi to an acupoint on the appropriate meridian.

The benefit of external chi is enormous in terms of convenience.

However, for more serious complaints the student should always consult a qualified Western M.D. before attempting any treatment, in addition to receiving advice from a doctor of TCM.

There are also chi applications through fingers and palm used in the martial arts. One is the One-Finger Art as applied by Master Hai Deng, whose hit at an opponent's acupoint may be fatal. This technique is also called *Dim Mak* (touch of death). It focuses the energy of the entire body on the index finger. When this finger is directed at certain acupoints *Dim Mak* can render the opponent's network of channels paralyzed or closed, thereby blocking his or her flow of energy and blood. Another application is through development of the Magic Hand, in which the palm is combined with the power of the five fingers, aided by intense thought concentration. This may immobilize someone else's movement—such as stopping his or her hand in writing or eating, and even stopping someone walking. This skill is called the way of immobilization, a martial arts skill of the highest form.

Notes

1. In Europe in the 1950s, Aristide Esser saw a Danish circus performer who could stand on his index finger.

10

Recent History of Chi Gong

The only solid piece of scientific truth about which I feel totally confident is that we are profoundly ignorant about nature.

—Lewis Thomas, *The Medusa and the Snail*

Breathing control gives man strength, vitality, inspiration, and magic powers.

—Chuang Tzu

Until the early 1980s, the existence of chi gong masters was considered to be a state secret in China. How the official Chinese perception of chi gong came to change throws light on the continuing ambivalence about its scientific status. In this chapter we will describe the political decision which thrust chi gong into the limelight, and go on to examine the direction of its present research and how psychic powers may relate to the practice of chi gong.

China's Psychic Debate

On March 11, 1979, in Sichuan Province's Dazu County, an eleven-year-old boy, Tong Yu, was discovered to be able to read with his ear. [1] With the newspaper report the news spread all over mainland China. Curious reporters from Beijing made special visits to

155

Sichuan, and their reports verified the story. The news spread beyond China. The reactions of most Chinese trained in modern Western science were predictable. Editors well-versed in dialectical material-ism were highly displeased, and sent their own reporters to Sichuan to interview Tong Yu. This time Tong Yu failed to display his psychic phenomenon. They announced that the news reports of Tong Yu's reading with his ear were false. These reporters and editors, who had been closed off from the Western world for thirty years, formed the vast majority. They banded together and made an attack charging that "A child's magic tricks should not be used to fool the world." Reporters who had seen the truth of Tong Yu's story with their own eyes were subjected to severe criticism. They soon realized that the only way to regain their credibility was to visit Tong Yu again to test and retest his ability to read with his ear. Tong Yu's psychic ability was demonstrated again and again. When still another group of antipsychic reporters visited Tong Yu, he again failed to display his psychic phenomenon. Tong Yu's psychic powers seemed to be affected by the attitudes of the reporters, and both camps held to their views.

Serious investigators of the paranormal know that psychic phe-nomena do not manifest themselves on command. It is accepted that when one's mood is a bit off, or one has not had enough sleep, or is hungry or sick, in a disruptive environment, or angry, psychic phe-nomena may disappear. On the other hand, when the subject is feeling psychologically secure, receives encouragement and praise, and is in a relaxed environment, psychic phenomena may appear. The prejudiced reporters who interviewed Tong Yu were suspicious; the way they talked may have frightened or intimidated Tong Yu. Also, if he was anxious or excited it may have interfered with any psychic effects.

Even when all environmental conditions are "right," psychic phenomena will not necessarily appear. Their coming and going without a trace is a cause for constant argument between believers and opponents. The mystery and inconstancy of the psychic phe-nomena finally led to a tremendous controversy in China.

Just when those for and against were heatedly discussing the Tong Yu case, fifty-two young people (aged four to twenty-five) from different provinces were discovered to possess exceptional human functions (EHF, also known as extraordinary functions of the human body). EHF is the Chinese designation for psychic or paranormal abilities. [2] After a year, tens of thousands of adults and children with psychic power were discovered in China! As a result, a psychic craze swept the country. Societies formed for the study of EHF sprang up all over China, and with that a huge national debate broke out. At one point, the partisans on one or the other side of the great debate included sixty-eight newspapers and magazines, forty-two educa-tional and scientific organizations, and fifty universities and colleges. Over one-half of all the radio and television stations in the country took part in the debate. Both the most notable representative of the pro faction, Prof. Qian Xue-seng, and the representative figure for the anti faction, Yu Guang-yuan, enjoy great fame in China.

Professor Qian, the most famous proponent of psychic phenom-ena in contemporary China, came to the United States to study in 1935, majoring in aeronautical engineering. Later, he earned a Ph.D. from the California Institute of Technology. During World War II he held the post of head of the Missile Unit of the Advisory Committee of the U.S. National Defense Sciences, and later that of Goddard Professor of Jet Propulsion at Caltech in Pasadena. After his return to China, he held the highest rank in science and technol-ogy as vice-president of the Academy of Sciences. He developed China's missile program, and it is entirely due to his efforts that China now possesses short-range, medium-range, and intercontinen-tal guided missiles. After the U.S. government sent Mr. Qian back to China, it is said that an official of the U.S. Department of Defense sighed regretfully, "Sending Mr. Qian back was the equivalent of

America's giving away four tank divisions to China." In 1970, fifteen years after Qian's return to China, the Chinese launched their first satellite, and in the decades since then China has successfully launched artificial satellites and tested many ICBMs (intercontinental ballistic missiles). As a result of China's experimental rocket launching program, a number of European countries have launched commercial satellites under Chinese auspices. In China, there isn't anyone who hasn't heard of Qian Xue-seng.

In January of 1981, Professor Qian published an article of over ten thousand words called "System Science, Thought Science, and Human Body Science" in Shanghai's well-known *Nature Magazine*. In July of the same year, he published another article, "Opening the Basic Studies of Human Body Science," affirming the value of chi gong and also asserting the existence of psychic phenomena.[3] He recognized these two fields as sciences and not the "magic tricks" which had been condemned by the opposing faction.

Yu Guang-yuan is a famous economist and the best-known opponent of exceptional human functions. Born before Mao Tse-tung, he has served as director of the Institute of Marxism, Leninism, and Thought of Mao Tse-tung, vice-chairman of the Chinese Academy of Sciences, and vice-director of Academia Sinica's Science and Technology Committee. During the battle over psychic phenomena, he published the first of a series of antipsychic articles ("Criticism of the Propaganda for 'Reading with Ear' in the Past Two Years") in the October 1981 issue of *Knowledge Is Power*, a well-known magazine in China. Of his seven planned articles, he only published three. Mr. Yu's book *Psi and its Variant: Exceptional Human Functions* did get published in 1982, but had little circulation, because the Chinese government, in an extremely rare move, forbade further discussion of psychic phenomena. Because the controversy between the two sides had become highly divisive for the nation, on May 13, 1982, the Central Propaganda Department issued a directive by the then general secretary Hu Yao-bang, ordering a halt to all further disclosure of psychic phenomena.

As a result, tens of thousands of proponents of psychic phenomena turned to the study of chi gong, because during the three years of uproar about psychic matters, a body of evidence showed that practicing chi gong often enhances psychic power. Since chi gong can build good health and cure illness as well as stimulate psychic power, it attracts even more interest than psychic power per se. This interest was all it took to provide a way out of the officially imposed silence on the proponents of psychic effects. In this way, within a year, chi gong research in China was flourishing.

What Happened to Chi Gong Research in China?

Throughout the three thousand years chi gong has been practiced in China, there have been periods when it has languished in obscurity. However, General Secretary Hu Yao-bang's political decision created the opportunity for chi gong to become familiar to China's one billion people and cure tens of thousands of patients, including cancer victims. Furthermore, the Chinese upsurge of chi gong also spread beyond China.

Prior to 1982 there had been official indications of the growing importance of chi in China. In 1979, the first national Qi Gong Scientific Research Seminar was held in Beijing, and the National Institute of Qi Gong (Beijing Qi Gong Institute) was established. On September 12, 1981, a National Qi Gong Research Society was formed under the sponsorship of the Traditional Medicine Association of China. After 1982 research intensified, and in 1988 scientists from all over the world participated in "The First World Conference for Academic Exchange of Medical Qi Gong" (to which we also refer in chapters 5 and 11).

Although in the past the use of external chi was not a routine part of the therapeutic arsenal of a doctor in traditional Chinese medicine, in Chinese medical circles the practice of chi gong has always been considered effective in curing diseases. Even during the reign of the Gang of Four (during the so called Cultural Revolution toward the end of Chairman Mao's life, approx. 1969–1976) when chi gong masters had been considered superstitious and backward, it is believed that people continued to find relief through chi gong for many illnesses, which proved resistant to conventional (Western or traditional Chinese) medical treatment. According to data culled from Chinese chi gong literature in recent years, chi gong has cured more than a hundred different kinds of diseases. As we discussed in chapter 4, many illnesses which can be treated successfully by acupuncture can also be treated effectively with chi gong, because they are based on the same therapeutic principle. Chi gong is especially effective for chronic conditions such as insomnia, headache, high blood pressure, etc., all of which can be cured without medication. As we reviewed in chapter 5, there have been cases of cancer cured by chi gong, and in many instances chi gong has reduced the patients' cancer symptoms and prolonged their lives.

Chinese scientists claim not only to have proved that chi gong can exterminate germs, but also to have manufactured several types of instruments, which are called chi gong therapeutic instruments (such as the Q-2 discussed in chapter 7), to imitate the external chi which is emitted by chi gong masters such as Lin Hou-sheng. These instruments are reported to have been used satisfactorily with patients, proving the existence of external chi. However, thus far there are many aspects of external chi that are still not understood. Although instruments can duplicate some of the physical (electromagnetic and infrared heat) aspects of the chi gong masters' outwardly directed healing powers, there is still no scientific way to model the informational aspects of chi.

Since chi gong can produce psychic phenomena, why hasn't it

been forbidden? It is because traditional Chinese medicine is recognized as a field of study by the Chinese government, and all aspects—whether acupuncture, herbology, massage, or chi gong—rely on knowledge of meridians, not on paranormal phenomena, to cure illness. Thus, using chi gong for health and medical purposes is legitimate. Proponents of psychic phenomena changed their orientation toward chi gong and psychic research, and there's nothing the government can do but keep one eye open and the other eye shut.

The Chinese government permitted research on chi gong abilities principally because these are considered to be scientific, whereas psychic abilities are unscientific, considered to be nothing but magic or deception. The difference in attitude toward the two phenomena is bound up in prejudice and subjectivity and lies in the distinction between innate and acquired abilities. Government officials felt that exceptional human functions claimed to be possessed by a person from the time of birth are most likely false, and should not be accepted by the public. Chi gong, on the other hand, is a functional ability which any individual can acquire through training. And any function which can be acquired by training is considered appropriate for scientific study. This is where prejudice and official subjective opinion presently stand.

Since 1979, Japanese, Malaysian, West German, British, French, and American scientists have visited China to inquire about chi gong. In July of 1983, a visiting team of medical scientists from Harvard University went to investigate the practice of chi gong (see chapter 11). They witnessed patients being anaesthesized by the emission of external chi, without any bodily contact, and could not provide an explanation.[4] One well-known and often quoted master is Lin Hou-Sheng, mentioned previously. On October 5, 1982, a group of Hong Kong scientists visiting the People's No. 8 Hospital in Shanghai observed the application of external chi in a surgical operation. They witnessed Master Lin Hou-sheng transmit chi by pointing his index and middle finger at an acupuncture point of the patient a few inches away. By doing so Master Lin spared the patient the need for a chemical anaesthesia. When the scientists left the hospital reporters asked them what they thought of the matter. Their reply: "What we saw with our own eyes was a miracle." During the past years Lin has repeated this kind of operation with satisfactory results each time. He can effectively anaesthesize people for as long as four hours by emission of external chi.

Professor Qian Xue-seng is deeply convinced of the scientific validity of chi gong. His wife had contracted an illness for which she underwent Chinese and Western medical treatments to no avail. Someone taught her to practice chi gong, and she was able to recover without the use of medication. Professor Qian has made great efforts to support chi gong research, appearing as a speaker at practically every national and local chi gong conference. His influence as a leading scientific figure has helped to sway popular opinion in the People's Republic of China to support chi gong research.

Regardless of Mr. Qian's support, the facts have proven that chi gong not only promotes health and cures illness, but also can be applied in sports training and other fields of national interest. In the past eight years, Chinese athletes have all been receiving chi gong training and have achieved outstanding results in numerous international competitions. During the Olympic Games in the U.S. in 1984, the well-known *World Journal* reported, "The athletes from Mainland China have quietly entered the arena using chi gong." It is especially noteworthy that Chinese women volley ball teams have defeated Japanese teams. American and Soviet intelligence officers soon learned about this secret and as a result the Soviet Union is now giving chi gong training to its athletes.

In education it is reported that practicing chi gong improves young adult students' academic work. Similarly, in the military it is said that the practice of chi gong enhances the soldiers' endurance, so that they can partake in longer marches and withstand conditions of severe cold weather.

Chi gong has risen in popularity in China and other parts of the world ten years after the acceptance of acupuncture,[5] but now it is receiving more attention than acupuncture in all parts of the world. At present, China has a national chi gong association based in Beijing as well as tens of thousands of local associations covering all county seats. Most medical service units engage in chi gong treatments, and many chi gong clinics have been established in all major cities. Three national chi gong periodicals are published in addition to many local chi gong magazines. Their total circulation is in the tens of millions. The Great Chinese Encyclopedia being compiled by the Chinese government includes an entry on chi gong study.

The Chinese maintain that chi is not a vague metaphysical notion; it is observable and testable. Many Chinese scientific facilities, including biological, physical, psychological, and medical institutions, as well as research institutes on nuclear energy, have proved that many kinds of energy are hidden within human bodies. The existence of human electromagnetic fields (also called human energy fields by the Research Section of Shanghai University) has been demonstrated and is being used in Western medicine. Chinese institutions using laboratory instruments have investigated chi gong masters. When they are generating external chi the following phenomena have been observed: infra-red radiation, static electricity, changes in magnetic fields, light waves, neutrons, beta rays, and two-way radiation of electromagnetic energy. Four scientists of the Chinese Academy of Sciences, Tao Jing, Wang Yong-hui, Li Yao-bei and Chung Wan-ji, investigated the existence of chi and issued a report entitled "The Qi Seen by Us." They wrote:

> It appears to us that qi is a much more complicated matter than we originally supposed it to be. Qi is probably a complicated organic combination of substance, energy, and message. At present, substance, energy, and message are studied separately in science. Scientists are very unfamiliar both in theory and in experiments with

what conditions will occur when these three produce effects at the same time.[6]

Since some manifestations of chi have been scientifically proven, and chi gong therefore has received the serious attention of scientists, we may anticipate its continued development. Researchers at various American universities have invited Chinese chi gong masters to deliver lectures, and some American doctors are learning to practice chi gong. We can safely predict that in the near future the study and practice of chi gong, together with acupuncture, will increase dramatically.

What Is the Connection Between Chi Gong and Psychic Powers?

How seriously should we take the claim that it is possible to produce psychic phenomena by practicing chi gong? We believe that, as with many other aspects of the human potential, every individual has a different aptitude, and attitude plays a primary role. It is claimed that some people display powers after practicing chi gong for a year; others have to practice as long as five years. Regardless of whether psychic power is stimulated by practicing chi gong or by external chi, the question remains, what is the cause of psychic power? Some Chinese researchers consider that after the human body energy (chi) is strengthened, the electric discharge of the cells becomes more coherent, and this brings about the emergence of psychic phenomena. Others feel that clearing the meridians and capillaries by stirring up the chi is the major influence. These partial, one-sided explanations cannot explain the emergence of psychic phenomena. The theory that attracts the most interest is that of the electromagnetic energy field. Whether in the human body or in the cosmos, electromagnetic (EM) fields play an important role. The strengthening of the EM energy field of the body would most readily explain the appearance of psychic phenomena, although the nature of the relationship between changes in EM fields and exceptional human functions remains mysterious.

Not only does the practice of chi gong help develop psychic powers, but it is said that in receptive people psychic abilities can also be induced by the application of external chi from a chi gong master. The method is quite simple. Selecting a sensitive person as a target, the chi gong master releases external chi to the relevant acupuncture points, which include the *dan tian, hui-jin, tangzhong, bai-hui, yin-tang* (midway between the eyebrows, the Gate to Heaven), and others. The external chi is applied at gradually increasing strengths at intervals of one or two days. However, one must bear in mind that even among those sensitive to chi not everyone can develop psychic powers and that such capabilities do not remain without practice. Stimulating psychic powers by external chi may provide a beginning, but the more suitable technique for acquiring psychic powers is one that relies on one's own continued practice of chi gong.

How does one select a person "sensitive" to chi? The simple method is to have the person extend a hand—the right if female, the left if male—with the palm facing upward while the subject relaxes. Then, a chi gong master releases external chi toward the subject's *laogong* point for about five minutes. If the subject experiences sensations of tingling, numbness, heaviness, or pressure, and if these sensations spread beyond the palms (as far as the fingers or wrist, or even through the whole body), then the subject is thought to be sensitive to chi. Often, sensitive subjects report a sour taste or heart palpitations. Another method is to release external chi toward the *bai-hui* or *dan tian* points, and see if "the feeling of chi" goes beyond these points. Still another method is to release external chi toward the *tangzhong* point and if the subject has the sensation of falling backward, he or she is said to be of the type sensitive to chi.

So far only the Chinese know the method of inducing psychic

powers with external chi. However there remain, even in China, strong opponents of the practice of chi gong and they focus their efforts on proving that chi gong is not efficacious in the treatment of disease and that its psychic powers are dubious. They have found support in the U.S. from the Committee for the Scientific Investigation of Claims of the Paranormal (CSICOP), whose representatives have recently traveled to China to disprove claims of exceptional human functions and chi gong masters' abilities. Professor Paul Kurtz, chairman of the Department of Philosophy at the State University of New York at Buffalo and the leader of their team, concluded: "In external qigong, a master can allegedly transfer an energy force. . . . They also claimed that they could diagnose a patient's illness by psychic means. When we tested both of these claims, we got negative results."[7] (See chapter 13 for a discussion of the CSICOP findings.)

In summing up, as to what the connection may be between chi gong and psychic powers, there is no clear answer at this time.[8]

Postscript On May 13, 1982, Communist China forbade further research into exceptional human functions using as a pretext the government's desire to stop the overheated debate regarding EHF. It appears, however, that there may have been an ulterior motive. Scientists in the Chinese army had purportedly proved that extrasensory perception (ESP) could be exploited for military purposes. In the meantime, students returning from the United States also reported that both the U.S. and Soviet governments had invested large sums of money in research on the use of psychic abilities for military purposes. They urged the Beijing government to pay heed to these developments.

It has been rumored that in 1963 the Soviets used a group of psychics to sink the American nuclear submarine *Thresher* in the Atlantic. We do not know to what extent this story is true. But ESP research units in China carried out experiments to test the strength of collective psychic power produced by a group of children with EHF. The experiments failed repeatedly. Once, however, when the timing appeared to be right and the children's minds may have been exactly synchronized, they were able to snap the trunk of a big tree. It is said that they also moved a large object from a distance. Although these experiments were top secret, many of the EHF researchers throughout China were too excited to keep this knowledge to themselves. They began whispering to one another. Soon the secret leaked out. This may have been the real reason for the government restricting research into exceptional human functions and putting an end to its public discussion.

In China it is generally known that practitioners of intensive chi gong may develop psychic powers. The number of people with innate psychic abilities may be few, perhaps one in a million, but there are now millions of Chinese learning chi gong. If even only one in a hundred chi gong students develops psychic powers, the number of people with acquired EHF will be ten thousand times more than those who have the ability from birth. ESP researchers the world over have speculated about this intriguing idea: Since China has the world's largest population and a great number of chi gong practitioners, it appears that the United States and the Soviet Union are at what could be a costly disadvantage in researching this mysterious and powerful phenomenon.

Notes

1. According to Dr. H. E. Puthoff in "Report on Investigations into 'Extraordinary Human Body Function' in the People's Republic of China," *Psi Research*, Dec. 1982, this phenomenon was also reported in the West as "eyeless sight" by Jules Romains, *Eyeless Sight* (Secaucus, N.J.: Citadel Press, 1978), and by Russian scientists as "dermo-optic perception," for example in L. M. Goldberg, "On Whether Tactile Sensitivity Can Be Improved by Exercise," *Soviet Psychology and Psychiatry* 2, no. 1 (Fall 1963). Paul Dong has also reported on this event in *The Four Major Mysteries of Mainland China* (Englewood Cliffs, N.J.: Prentice Hall, 1984).

2. Also see Dong, *The Four Major Mysteries.*

3. Also see *Psi Research* 1 (June 1982): 4–15.

4. Also see David Eisenberg, *Encounters with Qi: Exploring Chinese Medicine* (New York: Penguin Books, 1987).

5. This came about after Paul Dudley White, M.D., and a group of U.S. scientists witnessed acupuncture anaesthesia on their visit to China.

6. Tao-Jing, Wang Yong-hui, Li Yao-bei and Chung Wan-ji, "The Qi Seen by Us," *Qi Gong Magazine* Vol 1, issue 2, 1983.

7. Paul Kurtz, "The China Syndrome: Further Reflections on the State of Paranormal Belief in China," *The Skeptical Inquirer* 13 (Fall 1988): 49.

8. Great spiritual teachers have warned against the temptation of using meditation and exercise for the sake of obtaining psychic powers. To quote the Taoist Master Chao Pi Ch'en: "As the time passes demonic states will occur to the practiser in the form of visions. . . . He must compose his mind which must be clear within and without." Gopi Krishna, "The Aim of Yoga," *Psychic,* Jan./Feb. 1973.

11

Chi Gong Comes to America

One of the reasons Western science cannot measure Chinese science
is that unlike it, it is not unified science based on universal theory. . . . Our (Western) scientific paradigm cannot be a unit, not
only because its theoretical foundations preclude that, but also because it lacks . . . humane purpose . . . a goal [which] is to serve
human beings, as aspects of the whole of Nature.

—Bruce Holbrook, The Stone Monkey

Chi gong, tai ji quan (popularly known as tai chi), and martial arts are
all members of the same family. In ancient China, practitioners of
the martial arts always put chi gong first and foremost. They knew
that cultivating chi and stirring up chi was essential; insufficient chi
would lead to lack of strength and a weak striking force.

Tai ji, the best known expression of chi practice in the U.S., is the
most recent of the thousands of types of chi gong exercises developed
over time. But modern popular interest in chi-related activities found
its first expression in the kung fu movie craze initiated by the actor
Bruce Lee. These martial arts films show many incredible feats of
strength, skill, and endurance, which cannot be fully understood
without knowledge of how a chi gong master can manipulate chi
energy. For instance, only after finding the villain's "unguarded
point" can the hero defeat him. This is obvious to a hard chi
practitioner, who is accustomed to directing his chi and to guarding

169

his body against sharp objects. We find an analogy in Western mythology when speaking of one's Achilles' heel.

President Nixon's visit to China helped bring about the world-wide introduction to acupuncture, another use of vital chi energy. However, the increased acceptance of acupuncture as a therapy for painful conditions or as a substitute for surgical anaesthesia did not lead to an *understanding* of chi, which is needed to master chi gong. The reasons why the martial arts films or acupuncture were not able to draw attention to the underlying concept of chi is simple: Action movies are popular, no matter how unbelievable they are (think of James Bond movies), and the Western medical profession could only accept acupuncture for its results not for its theory. However, in the case of *tai ji quan*, which is also a true expression of chi gong, one might think that the unbroken tradition of teaching would have safeguarded the concept of chi. But, the fact is that the powers of chi became obscured and mystical until recently.

There was a famous *tai ji quan* master in China, known as Unbeatable Yang Lu-chan, who could knock down his opponent as soon as he released his force—probably what we now know as Empty Force (see chapter 6). This awesome force came from the Standing-On-Stake chi gong exercise. People felt that the power to "draw blood with one move" was too terrible, and for this reason they eliminated the Standing-On-Stake chi gong method from popular teaching, and focused on exercises sufficient to maintain health. In addition, *tai ji* was developed during the Ching Dynasty, 1644–1911 (this last dynasty was not of Chinese but of Manchurian, thus foreign, origin), which means that its teaching coincided with the exposure of China to Western influences. It is possible that because of this exposure, *tai ji* instructors, especially those outside of traditional areas of China, Taiwan, and Hong Kong, not only forgot about Standing-On-Stake, but also came to disregard the Chinese scientific underpinning: the knowledge of chi energy flow. In this

century, because of the Western (later Marxist materialistic) philosophy of China's rulers after the last emperor, the knowledge of chi
became esoteric. In 1929 the Chinese government went so far as to
forbid the practice of traditional Chinese medicine and tried to
replace it with Western medicine. For a while, chi gong masters had
to keep secret; their teachings were considered to foster superstition
or subversive doctrine. This situation prevailed through the early
seventies, until chi gong's recent revival.

Even though many teachers of Chinese martial arts and *tai ji*
outside of China have not emphasized chi gong, Chinese savants
(*shih*) and traditional chi gong masters have continued to provide
instruction with the chi concept as the fundamental teaching. In
recent years, since the rise of chi gong's popularity in China, martial
arts and *tai ji* instructors have also raised the banner of chi gong, and
they too now rely on chi gong as the fundamental teaching.

After chi gong became popular in mainland China, Taiwan, and
Hong Kong, it spread to Singapore and Japan. Within three years it
had traveled as far as Europe, Canada, and the United States.
Because the U.S. has the largest Chinese overseas community in the
West, it has a livelier group of chi gong enthusiasts. At present it has
spread to all large cities, but its greatest popularity is in San Francisco
and New York.

As soon as China's chi gong craze reached America, the *New York
Times* promptly carried a story, "A Traditional Chinese Therapy
Harnesses 'The Vital Force'." This immediately caught the attention
of the American public. The offices of the *New York Times* and
Chinese American associations in New York City received many
telephone calls asking for details about chi gong and inquiries about
where one could learn chi gong. As a result, in the year that followed
several places began to offer private lessons in chi gong. The number
of students has been increasing, and on October 24, 1988, the well-
known West Coast newspaper, the *San Francisco Chronicle*, published

another story, "Chinese Healing Art Focuses on Tummies." Hun-dreds of people made inquiries about this to San Francisco's China-town. By that time Paul Dong had already started a chi gong class in the Chinatown YMCA. It was one of the few classes which was taught in English and for this reason it attracted many American students. Once Dong asked them, "Why do all of you like chi gong?" They answered, "Because we all have caught the American disease!" At this everyone burst out laughing. "The American disease" refers to such chronic ailments as bad nerves and other symptoms of stress, sleeplessness, headaches, low back pain, high blood pressure, etc. Actually, people all over the world are prone to suffer from these ailments, and this may be the very reason why chi gong has become so popular all over the world. This statement is no exaggeration. The First World Conference for Academic Exchange of Medical Qi Gong, held in Beijing from October 10–13, 1988, was sponsored by the six countries of China, Italy, the U.S., France, Japan, and Australia. Twenty-six nations participated and there were 450 delegates. The event attracted worldwide attention. In chapter 5 we referred to some of the studies presented there.

We are pleased to report that a general interest in chi gong in North America is growing. Under the direction of Dr. Kenneth M. Sancier and Dr. Effie Chow of the East West Academy of the Healing Arts, Paul Dong taught a chi gong class for scientists in the San Francisco Bay Area. This class was scheduled to meet every Sunday for eight weeks starting October 2, 1988, and had seventeen partici-pants, including university professors, medical doctors, a pharmacist, and assorted people with advanced degrees. Under the sponsorship of the East West Academy of the Healing Arts the class covered such topics as What is Chi, The Mysterious Nature of Chi, Maintenance of Health, External Chi, and so on. Over half of the participants personally experienced the effects of chi. Because of this success, a second class was started on January 9, 1989.

On the first day of the class, Dong introduced six students from his YMCA class in order to demonstrate external chi and the power of chi. When he knocked his student Tom Chen back just by waving his hand at him (without touching him), most of the people on the scene apparently remained incredulous. Some called it a psychological effect, others considered it a hypnotic suggestion, while some condemned it as plain deception. Dong relied on the six advanced students to come every week to practice with the new students. This is because students who have practiced chi gong for a hundred days or longer already have a fairly strong electromagnetic body field, and thus can affect new students and allow them to feel chi more easily. As it turned out, by the end of the course, most of the new students were able to feel the presence of the chi field. One physically handicapped student, who was unable to move about freely, was asked to sit in the center surrounded by the other students in order that he be given the benefits of the chi feeling. He indeed felt the presence of the bioenergetic field. Another student, who had been most sceptical of Dong's demonstration of external chi, finally agreed on the existence of a body electromagnetic field. Yet another student, a professor at Stanford University, had been suffering from a pain in the foot for months. Dong gave him three external chi treatments, and he reported that his pain had significantly diminished.

A fourth student initially belonged to those who are not sensitive to chi, as measured by the methods described in chapter 10. However, by the end of the course he and five other students were going into spontaneous movement, a ceaseless moving around and shaking after having entered the quiet state (see chapter 8). This lends credence to the fact that anybody can develop chi energy flow through diligent practice.

The mystery of chi and its effectiveness in healing attracts people's interest the world over. The curious and research-oriented American public is no exception. In the past few years many reports on the mysterious nature of chi have appeared in the American print media. More importantly, the eighteen Chinese language newspapers published in the United States constantly report on chi gong. In San Francisco alone, there are twenty-two places offering instruction in chi gong. Chi gong students have formed three chi gong research associations on the West Coast. In San Francisco the Association of Chinese Qi Gong Health Exercises was established in 1986. Thus it appears that continued support for chi gong among the American public is assured.

Unfortunately, academic attempts to foster mutual respect and combined research efforts have not fared as well. An example is the history of repeatedly aborted medical chi gong research projects sponsored by the Sino-U.S. Qi Gong Health Sciences Development Center (SUQ). This effort was initiated by Robert Leeds, presently director of the US-China Peoples Friendship Association of Washington D.C. It began when in 1983, just after further publicity of EHF phenomena had been officially interdicted, a group of American researchers, including Drs. David Eisenberg and Herbert Benson from Harvard University Medical School, made "a formal medical expedition to China, especially to investigate Qi Gong therapy."[1] As described by David Eisenberg in *Encounters with Qi*, after some demonstrations of the effects of chi gong and evaluation of the data offered by Chinese Western-trained scientists as proof of the existence of external chi, both sides agreed merely to negotiations "for the testing of Qi Gong masters in American research laboratories."[2] Internal strife between Chinese researchers based in research institutes of Beijing and Shanghai, as well as divided opinion within the American delegation, interfered with open, complete, and unbiased presentation of all the facts. The visit ended inconclusively; to quote Eisenberg: "The burden of proof remains on the Chinese. Research to date cannot prove or disprove Chinese claims about Qi Gong."[3]

A follow-up visit organized by Leeds in 1984, during which Aristide Esser represented American medical research interests, brought about a more substantive, negotiated contract for research between the Beijing College of Traditional Chinese Medicine and the SUQ. This agreement included the exchange of scholars and initiation of specific projects, including research on cancer, hypertension, and the use of high technology instrumentation to measure external chi. However, beyond a 1985 return visit of a Chinese delegation, including chi gong masters, to several U.S. hospitals and medical schools, nothing came of these plans. A subsequent visit in 1987 of another American SUQ group led by Leeds, this time with many participants representing medical research interests, including Dr. James Young (AIDS and Public Health), Dr. Robert Sampson (AIDS and Traditional Chinese Medicine), and Dr. Fred Siegel (AIDS and Western Medicine), likewise produced only reports and proposals, without any actual research being initiated. The topic for this conference, "AIDS: East and West Approaches," was chosen by the Chinese. If AIDS is to benefit fully from acupuncture and chi gong practice (as it strengthens the body's immune mechanism) a program of research as was suggested by Dr. Sampson[4] must be pursued, but the Chinese medical interest of late seems to have shifted to the study of herbal treatment of AIDS.

The First World Conference for Academic Exchange of Medical Qi Gong in Beijing, August 1988, offered another opportunity for SUQ representatives to formulate research proposals. More than one hundred abstracts of scientific papers from many different countries were made available and medical scientists from the Chinese and Western traditions had the opportunity to exchange information freely during the four-day conference. Yet again, after this exchange had triggered a return visit by a Chinese group of officals and scientists in the spring of 1989, plans for US-China collaboration were not acted upon. Now, after the June 1989 suppression of intellectual and political dissidents on Tiananmen Square in Beijing, it seems extremely unlikely that official institutional agreements for scientific coordination of chi gong research will be implemented in the near future.

Now and then one hears of similar efforts to arrive at a mutually acceptable research protocol, and there may even be results from an occasional individual Sino-American collaborative study. However, we are not aware of additional insight generated by research to date that could lead to trusting cooperation between Chinese *shih* and Western scientists. And such a full exchange of ideas between those who understand chi from a lifelong study of its traditional expression and the most sophisticated minds in Western medical research is essential in order to unravel the fundamental nature of chi. We believe that comprehensive basic collaborative research projects can only come about when sufficient numbers of Western scientists become willing to accept the radically different worldview that animates traditional Chinese science.[5] And it is our opinion that this goal of mutual true-hearted synergistic research between the nations is best served by a personal acquaintance with the practice and benefits of chi gong, such as we have tried to foster in this book.

Yet, even with all these obstacles, chi gong is truly beginning to blossom in America and we hope that it will bring us deeper insights, good health, enjoyment, relaxation, peaceful sleep, and the prevention of headaches!

Notes

1. David Eisenberg, *Encounters with Qi: Exploring Chinese Medicine* (New York: Penguin Books, 1987), 199.

2. Ibid., 229.

3. Ibid.

4. See the manuscript by Robert Sampson, M.D., presented in Beijing: "Qigong Health Sciences and an Integrated Approach to the Treatment of AIDS," August 1987. It includes reference to an encouraging study on the effects of chi by Naomi Rabinowitz, "Acupuncture and the AIDS Epidemic: Reflections on the Treatment of Two Hundred Patients in Four Years," *American Journal of Acupuncture* 15 (January-March 1987): 25–42.

5. We cannot provide details here, but urge interested readers to consult, for instance, Eisenberg, *Encounters with Qi*; Bruce Holbrook, *The Stone Monkey: An Alternative Chinese-Scientific Reality*; and Manfred Porkert: *Chinese Medicine*.

12

Enjoyment of Life

The most beautiful experience we can have is the mysterious. It is the fundamental emotion which stands at the cradle of true art and true science.

—Albert Einstein, *What I Believe*

Chinese medical theory contains the proposition "The seven emotions damage the health." The seven emotions consist of joy, pleasure, love, anger, sorrow, hate, and desire (obsession). It is also said, "If you want to preserve health and cure sickness, just control the seven emotions." This is because the seven emotions frequently create instability of the spirit. If our moods are constantly disturbed by the seven emotions, our breathing and blood circulation will be congested, and from this disease may arise. Unfortunately, since we are bestowed with the senses of the eyes, ears, nose, and tongue, and a mind capable of thinking, there is no way to avoid the seven emotions damaging the health. The best an intelligent person can do is to control as much as possible the disturbances of these seven emotions, particularly avoiding the "demons of the mind," anger, sorrow, hate, and desire.

Overcoming the seven emotions is not easy. For this reason, ancient Chinese masters of health care created the method of silent sitting to preserve health, which is the present-day Relaxed and Quiet chi gong.

As stated earlier, there are three major kinds of chi gong—

177

movement chi gong, quiet chi gong, and combined movement and quiet chi gong. Each has its own uses, but quiet chi gong (silent sitting) is best for controlling the seven emotions, because quiet chi gong aims at entering a meditative state and calming the mind. It can eliminate distracting thoughts (the seven emotions) more easily, and if the mind has no distractions, the body will relax more easily. The combination of quiet and relaxation produces a comfortable feeling, a natural, wholesome form of enjoyment providing health and spiritual satisfaction greater than any pleasure attained through material possessions. Dong recounts:

My first chi gong instructor, Ms. Tian Wen Juan, doctor of traditional Chinese medicine, is one of the people I most admire (see also chapter 4). She had heart disease eighteen years before I met her. The doctors diagnosed her condition as very serious, with danger to her life if she wasn't careful. However, medicine could do nothing for her, so she chose to practice chi gong. After she practiced quiet chi gong for one year, her heart returned to normal. Thus, she was deeply convinced that chi gong is the best medicine, the best doctor, and the best treatment in the world. She made a determination to practice on a long-term basis. By the time we met, she was already beginning her eighteenth year of practice. Not only is she in good health, she also considers that practicing chi gong and entering a meditative state is one of the pleasures of life. One day, when we went out to dinner, she told me that she used to be a woman very concerned about clothes, food, shelter, and transportation. She wanted to wear pretty clothes, eat good food, live in a secure home, and get a car to go around in. However, her spirit was unhappy and she was very prone to disease. Today, she feels that there is no enjoyment more important than spiritual satisfaction. She said: "In the third year since I'd been practicing chi gong, I reached the highest stage of meditation, also known as 'the unity of person and heaven,' which means to disappear from one's senses, to seem to become a cluster of chi, to merge one's chi with the sky, earth, clouds, trees, and mountains."

I was highly interested by what she had said, because in a person's life it is difficult to have the chance to enjoy such natural pleasure. When we climb to the top of a mountain and look into the distance at the expanse of the earth, go to the beach and look at the ocean, or lie in a field and look at the blue sky and pretty clouds, don't we also feel exhilarated? Four years after that conversation, I became able through chi gong practice to enjoy that stage of meditation myself, but not every time. I have the feeling of freedom from my senses once out of every six times, and then my own body experiences that stage of "the unity of person and heaven." This is an indescribable joy. Money cannot buy such enjoyment. When I practice chi gong in the middle of the night and reach the highest stage, the self merges with the Milky Way, the cosmos, and the stars, and this feeling reminds me of a descriptive passage from a book in Western literature which I read as a child. Its overall meaning was: Suppose a person flew up into the clouds to heaven, and the bounds of the universe were in view, the galaxy was right there to see, the hordes of stars were sparkling, and the person could enjoy the night scenes of nature. It would be like entering another world, and the person would certainly feel great delight.

Although practicing chi gong and entering the meditative state is a supreme pleasure of life, very few people can achieve it. One must have enormous patience and persistence, gradually progress through each stage, and attain it only after a long time. Entering a meditative state means decreasing distracting thoughts, keeping a steady mind, and operating against internal and external stimulations to first weaken and then completely eliminate them. The level of the meditative state is determined by the amount of time spent. Entering the meditative state gives rise to a subjective condition of inexcitability and nothingness. The meditative state always becomes gradually deeper with the passage of time. Its manner varies greatly from one person to another, and even for the same person the feeling is not quite the same each time he or she practices chi gong. The beginning stage of the meditative state mostly entails a level head, a harmonious disposition, a peaceful mood, concentration of spirit, a decrease in distracting thoughts, and a fairly steady attention. At the next stage of practice, the mind quiets down more and there is a subjective impression of only one continuous, compact stream of awareness with which the mind is in tune. The mind and spirit are peaceful and the attention is focused. At a still higher stage of development of meditation, one has the feeling of imperturbability and nothingness, a stillness like water at rest, or a sense of lightly drifting aloft like wisps of clear smoke, or an impression of flowing as if riding on clouds, an intuitive perception which can be recognized but which is difficult to describe.

Owing to the relaxation of the whole body, the evenness of the breathing, and the emergence of the meditative state, the cerebral cortex is brought into a type of chi gong state. This has a beneficial effect on the organizational structures making up the meridians, the chi and blood, and the internal organs. As a result, the internal mechanisms of the body undergo all kinds of physiological changes. After entering the state of meditation, chi gong practitioners often have the sensations of a clear head, emotional ease, a happy spirit, and a steady mood. The whole body or some parts display sensations of warmth, lightness, looseness, and comfortableness, and as a result the chi gong practitioner is brought into a contented, cheerful, harmonious state.

The chi gong meditative state is a form of enjoyment, and this is also a key to activating chi gong's power. There must be positive encouragement toward eliciting the meditative state. A quiet environment with moderate light minimizes the stimulation to the cerebral cortex, and this is useful for the attainment and development of the meditative state. Practicing chi gong in a room at the right temperature and with fresh air, or practicing outdoors, often leads to a sense of exhilaration and a clear head, and has a definite positive role in bringing about the meditative state. A mind at ease, an optimistic attitude, and a steady, peaceful disposition are essential preconditions to correctly grasp the chi gong methods and implement its major points. Only by the discipline of practicing chi gong, and stepping up the practice gradually, is it possible, in turn, to achieve the effects of the meditative state. Firm confidence is also a basis of good chi gong practice. In addition, while practicing chi gong one should carefully stay away from mental burdens, psychological pressure, or impatience for results, in order to avoid stress to the nerves or excitement to the brain which would block entering the meditative state.

There are many methods of practicing chi gong to enter the meditative state, and the chi gong practitioner can select one way according to individual circumstances. The most commonly used methods for meditation gong include:

1. Focusing on the *dan tian* (the abdominal area below the navel, called *hara* in Japan and *svadhistana chakra* in India): Concentrate all attention on the *dan tian* while practicing chi gong. One can also focus on the natural rising and falling of the breathing.

2. Reciting to oneself: Select a phrase with an appropriate meaning, such as "Peace and quiet naturally bring good health," and recite it to yourself while in the process of practicing chi gong. One can also select a favorite short verse from a poem, speech, song, or prose work and recite it to oneself. After entering the meditative state, one will often forget about reciting to oneself; when distracting thoughts return one can use reciting to quiet the mind.

3. Counting breaths: Silently count how many times you breathe during chi gong practice, counting once every time you inhale, inhaling and exhaling once being counted as one breath. You can count from one to ten or one to a hundred and then start over again.

4. Visualization: Imagine a scene spread out before yourself, such as a glowing sunrise, a shining moon, clouds in an azure sky, green hills and beautiful waters, a vast sea, or fresh flowers and other plants. With the mind on these scenes, the concentration is focused and the mental state will be calm.

5. Guiding: Self-guiding involves lightly placing both hands in the area of the *dan tian*, moving the hand with the rising and falling of the breathing, and focusing the mind. This method not only can guide one into the meditative state, it also helps to settle down the *dan tian*. Another method is guiding by someone else, in which the guiding person's hand is placed in the area of the *dan tian* of the person practicing chi gong. This causes the attention to focus on the area of the hand contact or to become aware of its warmth, which induces entering the meditative state.

6. Internal focusing: This refers to forming a beautiful mental picture around the *dan tian* and focusing on the picture while practicing chi gong.

7. Focusing on internal organs (for patients): When some organ of the chi gong practitioner is diseased, the person focuses on the diseased organ. For instance, focus on the heart for heart disease, focus on the kidney for kidney disease, focus on the liver for liver disease, and so on. This method not only allows one to enter the meditative state, it also makes a definite positive contribution to the effectiveness of the cure.

You can try all of the above methods. After finding the method or combination of methods which works best for you, you should use that method only. Practicing chi gong and entering the meditative state brings about a sense of ease and comfort which, according to traditional Chinese medicine, leads to bodily health and longevity. Western scientific research tends to substantiate this with the observation that as a result of therapeutic hypnosis, a state akin to meditation,[1] the brain releases endorphins,[2] neurotransmitters that among other functions provide pleasure and ease pain, thereby promoting synergy of body and mind.

In conclusion, we can safely say that for those of us who are curious, or suffer from chronic treatment-resistant conditions, or who are getting tired of the rat race but find the modern ways of meditating insufficiently challenging, chi gong is an excellent way of learning to experience a different culture. More importantly, if the practice of chi gong contributes to a general understanding and willingness to consider facts from the radically different worldview of the Chinese, it may motivate modern Western science and technology, and especially Western scientific medicine, to learn and incorporate insights from the theory of traditional Chinese medicine.

Notes

1. For example, see the discussion in E. L. Rossi, *The Psychobiology of Mind-Body Healing* (New York: Norton, 1986), 182 ff.

2. These are the body's counterparts to the opiates found in plants, which for example in the case of opium, have been used to combat pain since time immemorial. See chapter 13 for further discussion of chi gong and endorphins.

13

Western Science and Chi

The extraordinary inventiveness and insight into nature of ancient and medieval China raises two fundamental questions. First, why should they have been so far in advance of other civilizations; and second, why aren't they now centuries ahead of the rest of the world? We think it was a matter of the very different social and economic systems between China and the West.

—Joseph Needham, *The Genius of China*, Introduction

From the perspective of modern Western science and technology there are several ways to deal with the manifestations of life energy, the Chinese concept of chi.[1] But, no matter where we turn, we will encounter stumbling blocks because of the differences in Western scientific and Taoist (traditional Chinese) thinking: Western research emphasizes form and function while Taoist learning looks for spontaneous natural harmony in process.

Where Westerners tend to look at appearance and substance, the Chinese are interested in relationships. Furthermore, as Bruce Holbrook has sharply brought into focus,[2] Western philosophy is preoccupied with an *absolute/fragmental* worldview—things should be defined precisely, in smaller and smaller fragments if possible, with little regard for the bigger picture. One could say that modern Western thinking is interested in an *ongoing analysis*. In contrast, according to Holbrook, Chinese philosophy attempts to fit everything into a *polar/complete* worldview—reality is seen simultaneously

185

as its polar opposites. This holistic way of seeing, where things are not separate but always part of a whole containing opposites, creates the big picture, the unity of all complementary appearances. The Chinese, from this perspective, may be said to be interested in an *ongoing synthesis.*[3]

It appears that the problems arising from an overly analytic orientation were already anticipated by the English philosopher and scientist Robert Hooke (1635–1703), one of the early secretaries of the Royal Society, founded in 1660. In those early days of modern Western science, Hooke outlined a two-phase plan for the advancement of science. First, there would be a phase of *increasing specialization* during which scientists would assemble vast quantities of empirical data. However, Hooke and his colleagues saw the possibility of becoming lost in specialized research, and therefore believed that after about three hundred years of this approach there should start the second phase of *unification,* when all the facts and parts of science would be integrated into a "complete system of solid philosophy."[4]

However, even as we begin to understand the need for unification of scientific data, the philosophical differences between Western analysis and Chinese synthesis still appear to rule the day. Therefore, initial Western reactions towards chi are often fueled by complete rejection—the suspicion that its manifestations are akin to magic, produced by quacks or charlatans, a result of outright deception. Subsequently, another reaction, strengthened by the rise of the human potential movement in the United States, has been to equate chi manifestations with psychic phenomena. To some extent this was influenced by recent public opinion in China, when so-called exceptional human functions were associated with the practice of chi gong, as discussed in chapter 10. Finally, there has emerged the contemporary deliberate and cautious outlook that chi is one of those yet unknown aspects of the mind/body interaction which the West is trying to explain by an integration of findings in quantum physics,[5] the brain sciences, and modern biology. It is the latter approach that offers hope for thoughtful integration, whereby we might begin to understand the results of thousands of years of Chinese synthesizing thought which produced the concept of chi.

Should Chi Be Considered Either Magic or Deception?

The main proponents of this view are the debunkers of paranormal phenomena, such as the Committee for the Scientific Investigation of Claims of the Paranormal (CSICOP). In 1988, a team under the direction of its chairman, Paul Kurtz, spent two weeks in China at the invitation of *Science and Technology Daily*, a leading Chinese scientific newspaper. Members of the six-person team, including the magician James (the Amazing) Randi, were "to appraise the state of psychic research and the extent of paranormal belief in China." Their report appeared in the summer and fall 1988 issues of *The Skeptical Inquirer*. Professor Kurtz writes about China:

> Paranormal beliefs have taken two main forms: First, many people claim to have special "psychic" powers. . . . The second area of belief that has enjoyed considerable popularity of late and seems to be growing is the use of Qigong to treat certain illnesses. . . . [it] is practiced throughout China in many traditional hospitals and institutes of medicine. A marriage of psychic powers and Qigong occurs in such places, as masters use alleged psychics to diagnose illnesses by seeing into a person's body without the use of expensive X-ray machines. During the cultural revolution, the Gang of Four attacked Qigong, but a movement is now under way to restore respectability to this "treasure" of Chinese culture.[6]

Following the reports in *The Skeptical Inquirer*, we summarize the results of the preliminary tests of various subjects who claimed to have special powers.

1. A test of a patient's movements purportedly resulting from the emission of external chi by a master, Dr. Lu, sitting in another room, "showed no significant correlation between the subject's movement and the Qigong master's efforts." Since the patient had moved simultaneously with Dr. Lu when they were in the same room, the report states: "We reasoned that in the context of their roles of master and patient, both knew what was expected of them. They both believed in the power of Qi to make the woman move, hence she moved. It was clear to us that Dr. Lu's movements *followed* those of the patient when they were tested in the same room."[7] (Italics in original)

2. A purported psychic, the younger sister of a chi gong master (names withheld at their request), failed to diagnose any of the physical conditions of four subjects.[8]

3. A test of two young women, who claimed to be able to see into a subject's body by psychic means to diagnose illnesses, gave results that could have been produced by chance.[9]

4. Several tests of "psychic" children resulted in either completely negative results or showed such evidence of cheating as tampering with seals used to secure containers, etc.[10]

Professor Kurtz concludes as follows:

One salient point emerges as we examine paranormal belief systems around the world: a belief-system does not have to be true to be accepted. . . . The placebo effect is also very strong: If people *believe* that something will make them better, this may contribute to some improvement in their condition.[11] (Italics in original)

We find the results of CSICOP's investigations of great importance for the exposure of obvious trickery and deceit. But we also believe that the reports incorrectly give a negative impression of chi gong as nothing more than a paranormal belief system or a placebo. As we have shown in chapter 1 and will review here, chi as a force/substance/process has several objective physical manifestations, which cannot be denied by saying that chi gong is only a belief system. As the remarks made by Professor Kurtz are not uncommon, we should examine some of their implications.

First, of course, we know that our assumptions, including those of modern science, are always part of a belief system. This point is also made in the pages of *The Skeptical Inquirer* itself. Dorion Sagan wrote, in an article on "Magic, Science, and Metascience," that: "both science and superstition partake of a magico-religious mode of thought for the simple reason that observations must be organized and the simplest working pattern proves to be the most expedient."[12] Second, we argue that chi gong as a method of improving health *should* be a belief system. Western scientific medicine too has discovered the importance of faith and cooperation in successful medical treatment. We also maintain that chi gong, regardless of the fact that some of its practitioners may make fraudulent claims or act as magicians, cannot be simply quackery or deceit as implied by Professor Kurtz.

The discovery of endorphins, for which Roger Guillemin and Andrew Schally received the Nobel Prize in 1977, may shed light on the role of belief in healing systems, and in turn on the role of chi gong. Endorphins are primarily known as morphinelike substances produced by the body to assist the brain in response to stress and pain. However, it is thought that endorphins may be master hormones that control all brain transmitters; since the same chemicals that control mood in the brain also control the tissue integrity of the body, endorphins are able to influence basic mind/body events.[13] In this sense some scientists have proposed that chi would exert its vital role through such chemicals as the endorphins, which would explain the dual substantive and informational effects that Drs. Xu Hong-zhang and Zhao Yong-yie have attributed to chi. Be that as it may, the placebo effect[14] shows that a belief system or suggestion/hypnosis have demonstrable therapeutic effects. Experiments demonstrate that the effectiveness of a placebo in pain relief can be reversed by the administration of naloxone, an opiate-antagonizing drug (that is, naloxone interferes with the beneficial effects of morphine and endorphins). Since the effect of a placebo, as proven in pain relief, is associated with the activation of endorphins, the quote from CSICOP's Professor Kurtz, that chi gong effects *merely* result from the individual's belief and the placebo effect, is at the very least shortsighted.

Should the Effects of Chi Gong Be Considered Paranormal?

Since the end of the last century, this question has been posed for any phenomena for which no ready explanation is available in terms of current knowledge about nature and mind/body interactions. Many of the observations dealing with paranormal phenomena (subsumed under the name "psychic research," following the establishment of the Society for Psychical Research in England in 1882), such as hypnosis, have subsequently become accepted as part of our mainstream knowledge. Other observations have been forgotten after they were found to be plainly wrong. Because of this constant change in what is considered to constitute psychic phenomena at any given time, research into paranormal phenomena tends to focus on hot topics, that is, observations that draw public attention. Such a topic was "reading with the ear," or dermo-optic perception, that captured China in 1979 and led to the exploration of the relationship between psychic phenomena and purported effects of chi, as discussed in chapter 10.

We can identify two specific areas of overlap between purported chi effects and hot psychic topics in the West: therapeutic touch and the human aura.

The concept of therapeutic touch, recently formulated by Professor Dolores Krieger,[15] goes back to the age-old practice of "laying on of hands," whereby the sick and handicapped experienced relief of their suffering when touched by their leaders, be these religious or the early royalty of England and France. Many of the contemporary faith healing meetings, often shown on television, feature this miraculous type of event. In terms of chi theory, its effects could be explained by the release of hard or external chi by the therapist or faith healer. Effects similar to the reported destruction of cancer cells by chi radiating from the hands of chi gong masters (see chapter 5) have been reported in North America as well.[16] In the daily practice of nursing, the beneficial effects of touching have been shown conclusively in such diverse applications as the alleviation of pain or the increase in hemoglobin values.[17]

Observations of the human aura, a luminous radiation around the body or parts of the body (as in the halos around the head depicted in religious art), have been known since antiquity. The phenomenon has recently been drawn into the field of physics by the development of so-called Kirlian photography. In 1939, the Russian Semyon Kirlian claimed that he could produce a photographic image of the aura of his hand when he placed a photographic plate between a metal electrode and his skin.[18] Since then, especially through the work of a Russian team at the Kirov State University of Kazakhstan, it was found that electromagnetic radiation of all living matter could be documented by this process of radiation field photography. The Russians claim that this reflects an energy body in addition to the physical body of atoms and molecules, which becomes visible if the living substance is placed in a high frequency electrical field. As we have seen in chapter 1, chi appears to be part of what we know as electromagnetic forces and chi masters report that they can see auras.

Thus it was to be expected that Chinese scientists have tried to use this method of photography to observe effects of chi.[19] We know of pictures showing external chi emanating from the index finger (see the reference made to a white substance, often seen in the chi gong practice for One-Finger Art, as described in chapter 9), but we do not know how this relates to Kirlian photography as it may be observed with the naked eye and therefore is not necessarily an electromagnetic phenomenon.

The possibility of photographing something resembling the mysterious aura, previously thought to be a purely occult phenomenon, as well as the examples of measurements of hard chi point to ways in which Western science and technology could explore the chi concept. We suggest that some of what are presently considered to be paranormal phenomena might be explored by (re)establishing the concept of a vital force in Western mainstream scientific thought.

How Can the West Study Chi as a Natural Phenomenon?

As we have argued, chi is not magic, nor is it merely a belief system or a product of hypnosis or suggestion. Chi, as the vital energy basic to mind/body interaction, should be part of general knowledge. Chi is part of our universe and our nature, and its research should be pursued in the basic and applied sciences.

We would like to look at the effects of chi as documented with present experimental methods of proof, as well as how these can fit within the developing theories of mind/body interaction in the West.

The manifestations of chi which appear to be most readily measurable with Western scientific instrumentation appear to lie in the clinical area and in the radiation of external chi. One clear and incontrovertible finding is the efficacy of acupuncture analgesia and anaesthesia, both in humans and in animals. Acupuncture is also widely used to treat illness in the U.S.; witness the fact that there are more than five thousand practitioners nationwide and that their treatments are reimbursed by several insurance carriers.

The use of acupuncture to ameliorate pain in 55 to 85 percent of the cases (that is, twice as often as with a placebo), is well documented. George A. Ulett, M.D., at Deaconess Hospital in St. Louis, Mo., has compared the analgesic efficacy of acupuncture (at points located by skin potential recordings) and hypnosis. He showed in controlled studies with twenty volunteers and twenty patients that electro-acupuncture (that is, the electrical stimulation of needles placed in the acupoints) worked equally well in poor as in good hypnotic subjects. This would mean that electric input given at specific points "was an effective agent for reducing experimental pain and that hypnotic susceptibility does not account for this effectiveness."[20] Also, Dr. Ulett found that acupuncture produced significant changes in brain activity as measured with the electroencephalogram (EEG) and sensory evoked potentials (SEPs), changes which did not occur with hypnosis.

Experiments also have shown that acupuncture treatment increases blood flow in body parts far removed from, but (according to the theoretical paths of the meridians), connected to the acupoints influenced. Mathew H. M Lee, M.D., at the Goldwater Memorial Hospital in New York City, a member of the New York State Commission on Acupuncture since 1973, has practiced acupuncture analgesia for many years. In 1983 he also began to study changes in skin temperature with acupuncture. One conclusion of these studies is: "[Acupuncture] induced a . . . longlasting, warming effect."[21] This would be in accordance with Western medicine's theory of the autonomic nervous system, which functions without the need for conscious recognition or effort by the organism. It is a system of motor and sensory nerves, supplying the internal organs (as well as blood vessels and glands) and connecting these for reflex purposes to all parts of the body via the brain and spinal cord. Thus it appears that the Chinese medical belief in relationships between points along the meridians and the body organs may relate to many autono-mous effects known in Western medicine, including Head's postulate of referred pain—for example, shortness in the supply of blood to the heart may show itself in pain radiating to the left little finger; gall bladder disease may first be indicated by a pain in the right shoulder.

Acupuncture is used routinely in veterinary medicine. According to Allen M. Schoen, D.V.M., president of the International Veterin-ary Acupuncture Society (IVAS), there are over 250 certified veter-inary acupuncturists practicing in the U.S. In September 1989, the IVAS held its Fifteenth Annual International Congress in Seattle, Washington. Countless articles and a textbook by Alan M. Klide and Shiu H. Kung, *Veterinary Acupuncture*, [22] have been published. If the effects of chi are solely based on belief systems, as was suggested by members of the Committee for the Scientific Investigation of Claims of the Paranormal (CSICOP), one might ask whether these investigators think that animals share the *belief systems* of humans!

Returning to human clinical applications, operations using nothing but the anaesthesia provided by the external chi from the fingers of a chi gong master were described in chapters 1 and 7. The least we should conclude from these clinical observations is that the underlying principle of both acupuncture and chi gong, the regula-tion of chi through its body channels (the twelve meridians), must have some material basis to be capable of replacing chemical and other methods of anaesthesia and pain control.

Acceptance of a material basis for the concept of circulating chi has also been strengthened by the measurement of variations in human skin resistance along the acupuncture meridians and around acupoints. In the early seventies Robert O. Becker, M.D., began his studies on the theory that acupuncture meridians were electrical conductors which sent messages to the brain. He proved that the expected lower skin resistance over the acupoints (which would be acting as amplifiers for the electrical current flowing through the meridians) could be shown to exist in half of the acupoints tested with the sensitive electrode he designed. Thus he felt "that at least the major parts of the acupuncture charts had . . . an objective basis in reality."[23]

We believe it is possible to conclude from all these findings that chi as a substance/force/messenger could well be hypothesized to exert its function via the autonomous nervous system and the release of neuropeptides, following the meridian system or the previously mentioned "psychosomatic network," envisaged by Candace Pert and co-workers.[24]

To the clinical evidence for a material basis of chi we add the measurements of a whole range of physical manifestations of external chi described in chapter 1, and conclude that chi is indeed a natural phenomenon, even if occidental science has thus far been unable to incorporate its existence.

As to possible Western research areas which have been considered in terms of accommodating chi effects, we can mention (self-)hypnosis or suggestion, meditation or (progressive) relaxation, and the emerging field of psychoneuroimmunology. Not one of these domains of knowledge has been able to accommodate all the diverse claims and findings regarding chi, but each has contributed toward further understanding.

Observation of the effects of chi have been attributed to suggestion, and the therapeutic effects of chi gong to self-suggestion or self-hypnosis. The role of suggestion and hypnosis in healing is an ancient and venerable one. Healers in primitive cultures (shamans, as they were called in Siberia, medicine men, witch doctors, etc.), use self-hypnosis to contact the spirit world and thereby increase their healing powers. Knowledge of this traditional practice accounts for the claims that the ancient art of chi gong is nothing but self-suggestion and the purported effects are caused by trickery on the part of practitioners, so that the observer is lulled into illusory findings. There is no doubt that suggestion and hypnosis can account for many strange or paranormal phenomena, as mentioned in chapter 2 regarding mind/body interactions. Certainly, reduction of pain is often readily accomplished by suggestion or hypnosis, as are feelings of well-being and health. However, as we have discussed above, acupuncture brings about different physiological changes than hypnosis and we cannot explain how it would work in animals, nor could suggestion account for the measurements of external chi. Also, the heightened awareness and razor-sharp reflexes exhibited by martial arts masters who have acquired their capabilities through chi gong, are not indicative of functioning under the influence of subconsciously induced hypnosis.[25]

The practice of induced relaxation as well as meditation, which is an acknowledged part of the practice of chi gong, has been considered as sufficient cause for the purported effects of chi. Again, meditation has roots going back to ancient times and is practiced in one form or another in practically all known cultures.[26] One well-known physician, who has had opportunity to study different types of meditation in different cultures and under different conditions, is Herbert Benson of Harvard Medical School. As he initially viewed it,[27] meditation (and yoga, prayer, hypnosis, etc.) was nothing but a "relaxation response," which is "an integrated hypothalamic response resulting in a generalized decreased sympathetic nervous system activity."[28] In his opinion, all the purported effects of meditation result from the simple practice of relaxation for ten to twenty minutes once or twice a day: Sitting quietly, breathing naturally, and with each exhalation using a repetitive thought, idea, or word (e.g., the well-known mantra om mani padme hum of yoga) enables disregard for any other content of the mind during this exercise. Benson proposed in 1983 that chi gong begins with the relaxation response[29] and from Benson's own writing it does not appear that the assumption of chi energy is needed to explain observations of purported chi effects. Benson later added the "faith factor" to the simple ingredients which provide for the relaxation response:

It has to be done "in the context of a deeply held set of personal, religious, or philosophical beliefs."[30]

We have referred above to the role of belief (faith) in any response to a healing practice when rejecting the dismissive remarks Professor Kurtz made of chi gong after CSICOP investigated paranormal phenomena in China. Regarding Professor Benson's feeling that chi gong can be subsumed under the relaxation response, even with the addition of a faith factor, we likewise maintain that his explanations deal only with a few of the effects of chi. We might say that such explanations are necessary but not sufficient in the case of chi. Our immediate reason for making this statement is that only the Chinese theory of chi can explain the application of acupuncture and external chi in anaesthesia and pain control, especially in animals. There is no doubt that meditation (and therefore Benson's relaxation response) is an integral aspect of chi gong, but physiological responses to meditation do not explain adequately the whole cloth which the theory of chi weaves for such widely divergent and successful clinical practices as acupuncture, the application of external chi and herbology.

Finally, there is the new discipline of psychoneuroimmunology, for which there are no ancient precursors as there were for modern hypnosis and meditation. In the past few years psychoneuroimmunology has come into vogue as a medical term referring to studies of the interactions between the mind, the body, and the immune system in health and disease. The relationship between stress, depression, and failure of the immune system in disease has been clarified in many studies. One of the diseases in which the mind/body interaction expressed through the immune system seems to play a major role is cancer. In chapter 5 we have referred to the importance of a positive attitude and mutual feelings of support in a patient's fight against cancer.[31] It has been shown that the hormones our body produces in response to stress decrease immunological defenses, and that in contrast positive feelings, laughter, faith, and the will to live all contribute to increased function of our immune system.[32]

The Future of Western Scientific Medicine and Chi

We could point to many more relationships between our mental attitudes, bodily functions, and abilities to withstand or prevent disease. But here we only want to emphasize that the concept of chi in the context of ancient Chinese observations appears to fit the psychoneuroimmunological findings as well as our earlier observations regarding (self-)hypnosis and meditation. Noting chi gong's effect on cancer or chronic debilitating disease, or the healing abilities of those who have mastered the movement of chi in the practice of traditional Chinese medicine, one cannot help but be impressed by the similarities with aspects of the healing process in Western scientific medicine observed in recent research.

It is clear that Western scientists will benefit by taking into account bioenergetic forces (if not the whole concept of chi) when thinking of research experiments within their disciplines. Willingness to learn firsthand about the vital force of chi is shown by those scientists and engineers who have started practicing chi gong. Their personal acceptance of a heretofore unknown energy may help revolutionize Occidental knowledge.

We end this book with the speculation that, in terms of psychoneuroimmunology, chi gong appears to offer a way to mix a cultivation of mental attitude with a strengthening of bodily functions in order to provide a balanced flow of matter/energy that informs our immune system. Achieving that synergic process, according to ancient Chinese wisdom, is elucidated by the concept of chi. If the Chinese are right in their polar/complete concept of a flow of life energy through its own meridian system, complementing the flow of blood through the cardiovascular system, our acceptance of chi is the essential step on the way to health.

Notes

1. Aristide Esser attempted to review challenges posed by chi to the West during a 1984 meeting between representatives of the Sino-U.S. Qi Gong Health Sciences Development Center and staff of the Beijing College of Traditional Chinese Medicine. See Aristide H. Esser, "The Use of Advanced Western Medical Science and Technology in the Study of Qi," *Chinese Culture* 26 (March 1985): 37–45.

2. Bruce Holbrook, *The Stone Monkey: An Alternative Chinese-Scientific Reality* (New York: William Morrow, 1981).

3. The term *synthesis* in this context does not refer to polar opposites merging into a higher unity so as to be separately indistinguisable. (This form of synthesis was one of the goals of the dialectical process identified by the philosopher G. W. Hegel [1770–1831] in his development of the Absolute. The method may be simply described as positing something as a thesis, then realizing that it can only be truly defined by taking other aspects or its opposite into account (antithesis), and finally arriving at the explicit recognition that thesis and antithesis are related on a higher level of objective truth: synthesis.) To understand ongoing process, which Chinese philosophy favors in the spirit of synthesis, we might consider the psychological concept of integration: a mental combination of opposites in which their characteristics remain distinguishable. Something similar is at work when a physicist explains the theory of light: While constantly remaining aware of light's incompatible characteristics, it is possible to refer simultaneously to light as a particle and as a wave.

4. We are grateful to Donald Benson who brought to our attention the material in Alice M. Hilton, ed., *The Evolving Society* (New York: Institute for Cybercultural Research, 1966), 10. Benson used this insight as one of the arguments for his further development of the concept of synergy, in D. Benson: *Guidebook to the universe: Some contributions to the theory and practice of Synergy* (Belhaven, NC: The Synergy Project, 1977).

5. Many contemporary physicists have paid tribute to the influence of Chinese thinking on their theories. After all, physics is one of the sciences which for years has accepted irreconcilable explanations for the same phenomenon. For instance, the dual theory of light shows the value of the Chinese principle of complementarity and the notion that truth need not be absolute.

6. Paul Kurtz, "Testing Psi Claims in China," *The Skeptical Inquirer* 12 (Summer 1988): 364–65.

7. Paul Kurtz et al., Ibid., 368.

8. Ibid., 370.

9. Ibid., 371.

10. Ibid., 372–74.

11. Paul Kurtz, "The China Syndrome," *The Skeptical Inquirer* 13 (Fall 1988): 49.

12. Dorion Sagan, "Magic, Science, and Metascience," *The Skeptical Inquirer* 11 (Spring 1987): 278.

13. Candace Pert and colleagues have proposed that neuropeptides (a class of chemicals to which endorphins belong) function in a "previously unrecognized psycho-somatic network."—E. L. Rossi, *The Psychology of Mind-Body Healing* (New York: Norton, 1986), 182. As they put it: "Neuropeptides and their receptors thus join the brain, glands, and immune system in a network of communication between brain and body."—C. Pert et al. in *The Journal of Immunology* 135 (1985): 820s–26s.

14. Placebo: from the Latin, meaning "I shall please." In modern medicine it refers to an inert, harmless substance that may be used when treatment is needed while the nature of the condition to be treated is unclear. In scientific drug testing a placebo is used to make sure that any therapeutic result is not caused by the patient's simple act of taking a medication or the natural wish of every doctor that a medicine may prove successful. The placebo effect shows that even in drug tests with inactive substances (or in analogous treatments with ineffective procedures) there is a 20 to 40 percent positive response! This means a placebo or any procedure that influences the mental state of the patient is obviously able to trigger actual changes in the body, such as the release of endorphins.

15. Dolores Krieger, *The Therapeutic Touch: How to Use Your Hands to Help or Heal* (Englewood Cliffs, N.J.: Prentice Hall, 1979).

16. For instance, the work of Bernard Grad, "Some Biological Effects of the 'Laying-on-of-Hands': A Review of Experiments with Animals and Plants," *Journal of the American Society of Psychical Research* 59 (1965): 95–127.

17. See for example D. Krieger, *Living the Therapeutic Touch* (New York: Dodd Mead and Co., 1987). For similar results after chi gong see chapter 8 in this book.

18. Nikola Tesla, the great inventor and rival of Thomas Edison, around the turn of the century used his invention, the Tesla coil, to make photographs of light emanating from the body.

19. For a brief history of Kirlian photography see Sheila Ostrander and Lynn Schroeder, "Science Probes the Energy Body," chapter in *Psychic Discoveries Behind the Iron Curtain* (Englewood Cliffs, N.J.: Prentice Hall, 1970).

20. Bruce Pomeranz and Gabriel Stux, eds., *Scientific Basis of Acupuncture* (New York: Springer-Verlag, 1989), 194.

21. See Matthew Lee and Monique Ernst, "Clinical and Research Observations on Acupuncture Analgesia and Thermography," in *Scientific Bases of Acupuncture*, ed. Bruce Pomeranz and Gabriel Stux (New York: Springer-Verlag, 1989), 167.

22. Alan M. Klide and Shiu H. Kung, *Veterinary Acupuncture* (Philadelphia: Univ. of Pennsylvania Press, 1987).

23. See Robert Becker and Gary Selden, *The Body Electric: Electromagnetism and the Foundation of Life* (New York: William Morrow, 1985), 236.

24. C. Pert et al. in *The Journal of Immunology* 135 (1985): 820s–26s. See note 13, above.

25. According to Professor J. Walker, martial arts training "can be dangerous to you and your opponent." The basic physics of forces rotating and torques shows how important it is to make split-second decisions about even the slightest of movements. J. Walker, *Roundabout: The Physics of Rotation in the Everyday World* (New York: W. H. Freeman, 1979).

26. For a comprehensive overview of meditation see John White, ed., *What Is Meditation?* (New York: Anchor/Doubleday, 1974); and Daniel Goleman, *The Meditative Mind* (Los Angeles: Tarcher, 1988).

27. Herbert Benson came to this view as a result of research by R. K. Wallace reported in *Science*, 27 March 1970. Benson and Wallace later coauthored an article in *Scientific American*, February 1972.

28. Herbert Benson in *Integrative Psychiatry* 1 (1983): 15–18; and *Trends in Neuroscience*, July 1983, 281–84.

29. David Eisenberg, *Encounters with Qi: Exploring Chinese Medicine* (New York: Penguin Books, 1987), 221.

30. Herbert Benson, *Your Maximum Mind* (New York: Random House, 1987), 6–7.

31. A recent American study showed that group therapy support combined with lessons in self-hypnosis decidedly increased cancer survival in women with breast cancer over a ten-year period. D. Spiegel, M.D., of Stanford Univ. Medical School, as reported at the 1989 Annual Meeting of the American Psychiatric Association.

32. See for example N. Cousins, *Anatomy of an Illness* (New York: Norton, 1979) and *Head First: The Biology of Hope* (New York: Dutton, 1989); M. S. Gazzaniga, *Mind Matters* (Boston: Houghton Mifflin, 1988); R. M. Restak, *The Mind* (New York: Bantam, 1988); E. L. Rossi, *The Psychology of Mind-Body Healing* (New York: Norton, 1986); B. S. Siegel, *Peace, Love, and Healing* (New York: Harper and Row, 1989).

RECOMMENDED READING

John Blofeld. *Taoism, the Quest for Immortality*. London: Unwin Paperbacks, 1979.

An introduction to Tao, the way, to whose practice chi gong belongs as the cultivation of vital energy.

Cho Ta-hung. *Knocking at the Gate of Life and Other Healing Exercises from China*. Emmaus, Pa.: Rodale Press, 1985.

This official handbook of the People's Republic of China is translated by Dr. Edward C. Chang. It offers an overview of many therapeutic self-help practices related to chi without referring to the underlying traditional science. It may be considered a modern counterpart to the tradition-based book by Dr. Siou listed below.

Paul Dong. *The Four Major Mysteries of Mainland China*. Englewood Cliffs, N.J.: Prentice Hall, 1984.

Born in mainland China, the Oakland-based author reports on China's fascination with UFOs, psychic phenomena, chi gong, and Wildman, China's equivalent of Bigfoot.

David Eisenberg. *Encounters with Qi: Exploring Chinese Medicine*. New York: Penguin Books, 1987.

Experiences of a Chinese speaking American M.D. who studied and did research in mainland China.

Bruce Holbrook. *The Stone Monkey: An Alternative Chinese-Scientific Reality.* New York: William Morrow, 1981.
    A superb introduction to concepts behind the practice of traditional Chinese medicine. The author is an American anthropologist who apprenticed himself to a Chinese savant and medical doctor (*shih-fu*).

Lao Tzu. *Tao Te Ching: The Book of Perfectibility.* London: Concord Grove Press, 1983.
    The classic text by one of the world's greatest philosophers discussing the wisdom of the Tao (see also Blofeld, above). In this edition there is a foreword on "Choosing the Tao" by Rhagavan Iyer.

Manfred Porkert. *The Theoretical Foundations of Chinese Medicine: Systems of Correspondence.* Cambridge Mass.: M.I.T. Press, 1974.
    A basic text by a German sinologist.
————. *Chinese Medicine: Its History, Philosophy and Practice, and Why It May One Day Dominate the Medicine of the West.* New York: William Morrow, 1988.
    Lucid and authoritative, includes a systematic comparison of the Western and Chinese medical paradigms, providing the basis for their complemental co-existence.

Lily Siou. *Ch'i Kung: The Art of Mastering the Universal Life Force.* Rutland, Vt.: Charles E. Tuttle, 1975.
    The author, former dean at the Hong Kong Christian College, describes many exercises in pictures and provides synopses of their ancient theoretical background. The book is a counterpart to the Western approach of Cho's book listed above.

Ralph G. H. Siu. *Chi: A Neo-Taoist Approach to Life.* Cambridge, Mass.: M.I.T. Press, 1974.
    A thoughtful book by a Western-trained Chinese biochemist, pointing to obvious shortcomings in the modern Western scientific view of life.

The Skeptical Inquirer. The journal of the Committee for the Scientific Investigation of Claims of the Paranormal.
    Specializes in debunking psychic phenomena. The issues of summer and fall 1988 report on an investigation of chi claims during a trip to China.

Robert Temple. *The Genius of China: 3,000 Years of Science, Discovery, and Invention*. New York: Simon and Schuster, 1986.

An excellent overview of the accomplishments of traditional Chinese science by the director of the world-famous Needham Institute, Cambridge University.

Marcello Truzzi. "Chinese Parapsychology: A Bibliography of English Language Items," in *Zetetic Scholar* 10 (1982): 143–45, and 12/13 (1987): 58–60.

An essential overview of the available literature, especially important as background for chapters 10 and 13 of this book.

I. Veith, trans. *The Yellow Emperor's Classic of Internal Medicine*. 2nd ed. Berkeley, Calif.: Univ. of California Press, 1972.

INDEX

(**bold** page numbers indicate definition or explanation of the subject)